A VISIT TO HOSPITAL

Gillian Mercer and Peter Dennis

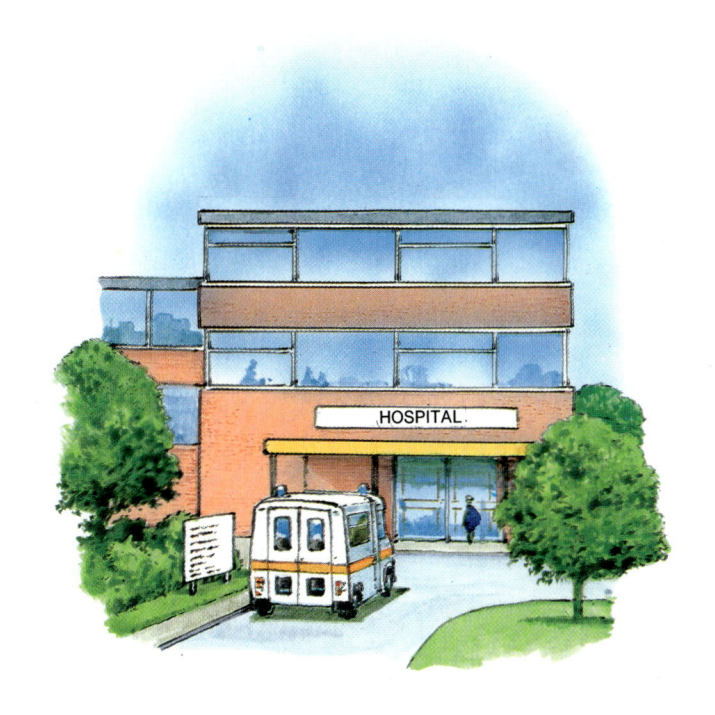

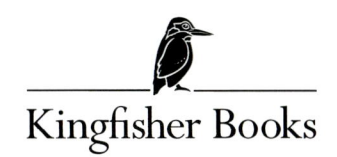

Kingfisher Books

Educational advisers: Mary Jane Drummond,
Cambridge Institute of Education, Cambridge
Iris Walkinshaw, Headteacher, Rushmore Infants School, London

Technical advisers: Hazel Foale (Ward Sister)
Guy's Hospital, London; Pauline Shelley and Jan Date,
National Association for the Welfare of Children
in Hospital (NAWCH); Gay Oliver (Physiotherapist)
Moreton-in-Marsh Hospital

The author, illustrator and editor would also like to thank
Patty Preston and the nurses and other staff at
King's Mill Hospital, Sutton-in-Ashfield, for their generous
help in the preparation of this book.

Kingfisher Books, Grisewood & Dempsey Ltd,
Elsey House, 24–30 Great Titchfield Street,
London W1P 7AD

This reformatted edition first published in 1992
by Kingfisher Books
10 9 8 7 6 5 4 3 2

Originally published in 1988 as *Stepping Stones 456: Inside a Hospital*
by Kingfisher Books

© Grisewood & Dempsey Ltd 1988, 1992

All rights reserved. No part of this publication may be
reproduced, stored in a retrieval system or transmitted by
any means electronic, mechanical, photocopying or otherwise,
without the prior permission of the publisher.

British Library Cataloguing in Publication Data
A catalogue record for this book is available
from the British Library.

ISBN 0 86272 955 6

Edited by Vanessa Clarke
Editorial assistant: Camilla Hallinan
Cover designed by Pinpoint Design Company
Handwriting by Jack Potter
Phototypeset by Southern Positives and Negatives (SPAN),
Lingfield, Surrey
Printed and bound in Spain

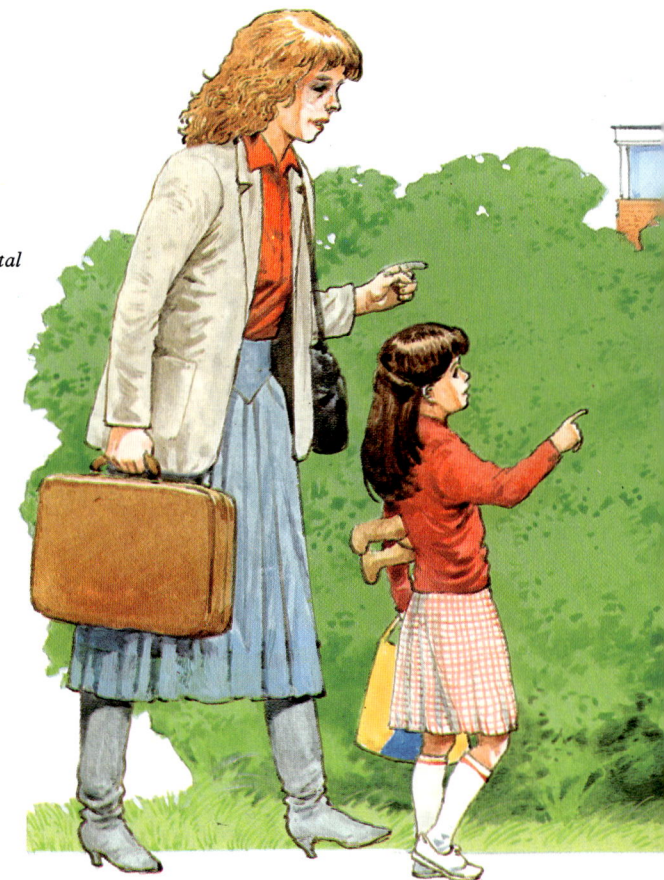

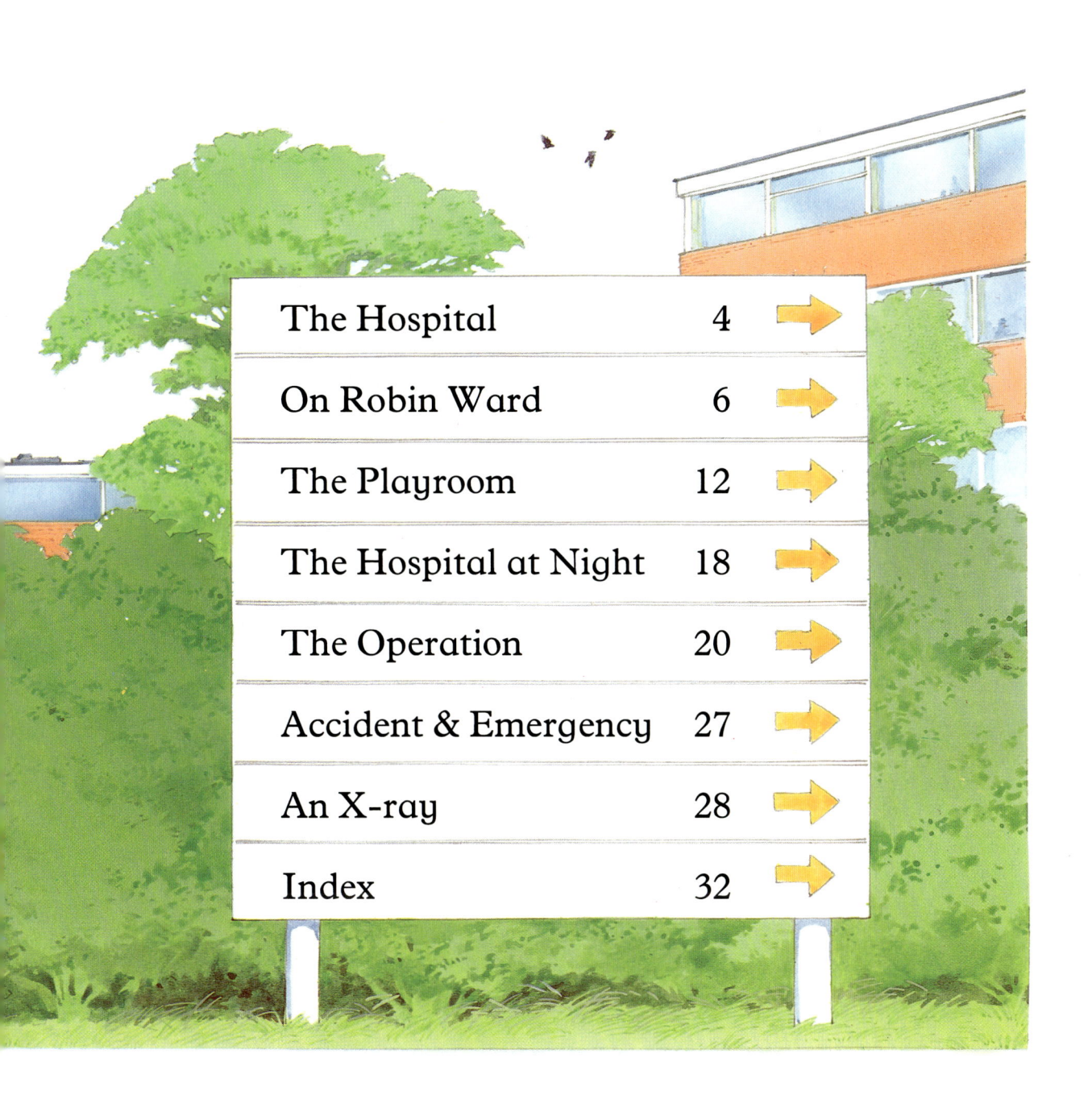

The Hospital	4
On Robin Ward	6
The Playroom	12
The Hospital at Night	18
The Operation	20
Accident & Emergency	27
An X-ray	28
Index	32

The Hospital

Here is the hospital. The people going through the doors have come because they are ill and the nurses and doctors will help them to get better. They are called patients while they are in hospital. Sometimes their families come with them too.

The first person the patients meet is Fred, the head porter, at Reception. He helps them to find the department they want. The hospital is like a large shop with many different departments. There are Operating Theatres where people have operations, X-ray Rooms where pictures are taken of people's insides, Maternity Units where babies are born, and rooms called Wards where patients rest in bed and sleep.

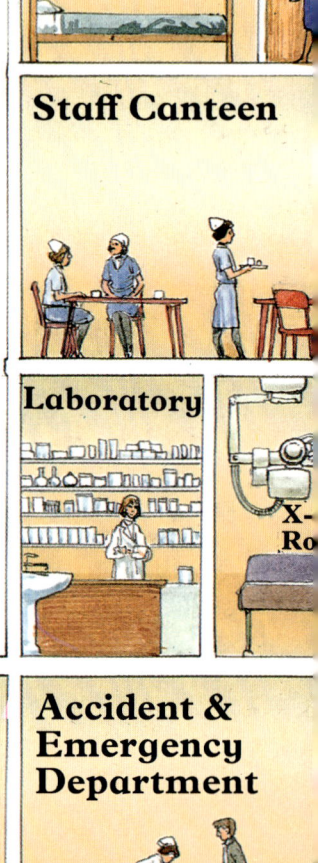

Parents' Room

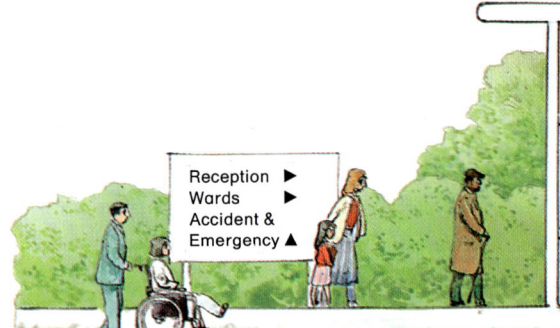

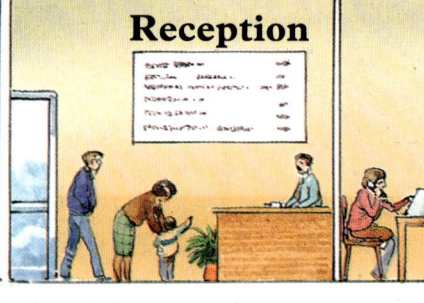

Staff Canteen

Laboratory

X-Ro

Reception ▶
Wards ▶
Accident &
Emergency ▲

Reception

Accident & Emergency Department

Playroom

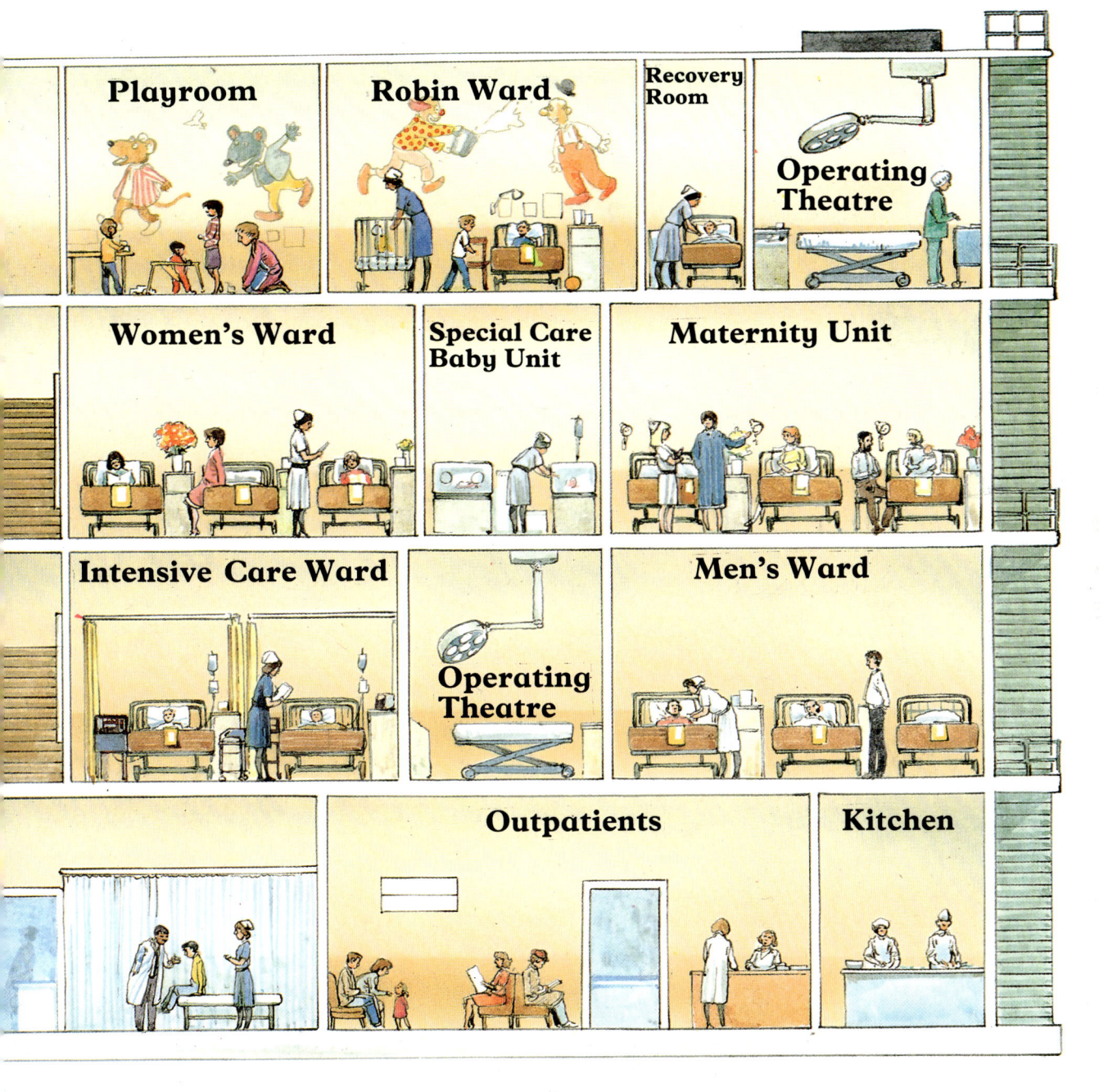

Robin Ward

Recovery Room

Operating Theatre

Women's Ward

Special Care Baby Unit

Maternity Unit

Intensive Care Ward

Operating Theatre

Men's Ward

Outpatients

Kitchen

On Robin Ward

This is Robin Ward for children. Sister Carole is saying hello to Amy who has just arrived. Amy has come to hospital because she has a hernia which makes her tummy hurt. She will be having an operation to put it right. Sister Carole is in charge of the Ward. Martin has to stay in bed because his leg is broken, but everyone else is up.

Hello, You must be Amy.

7

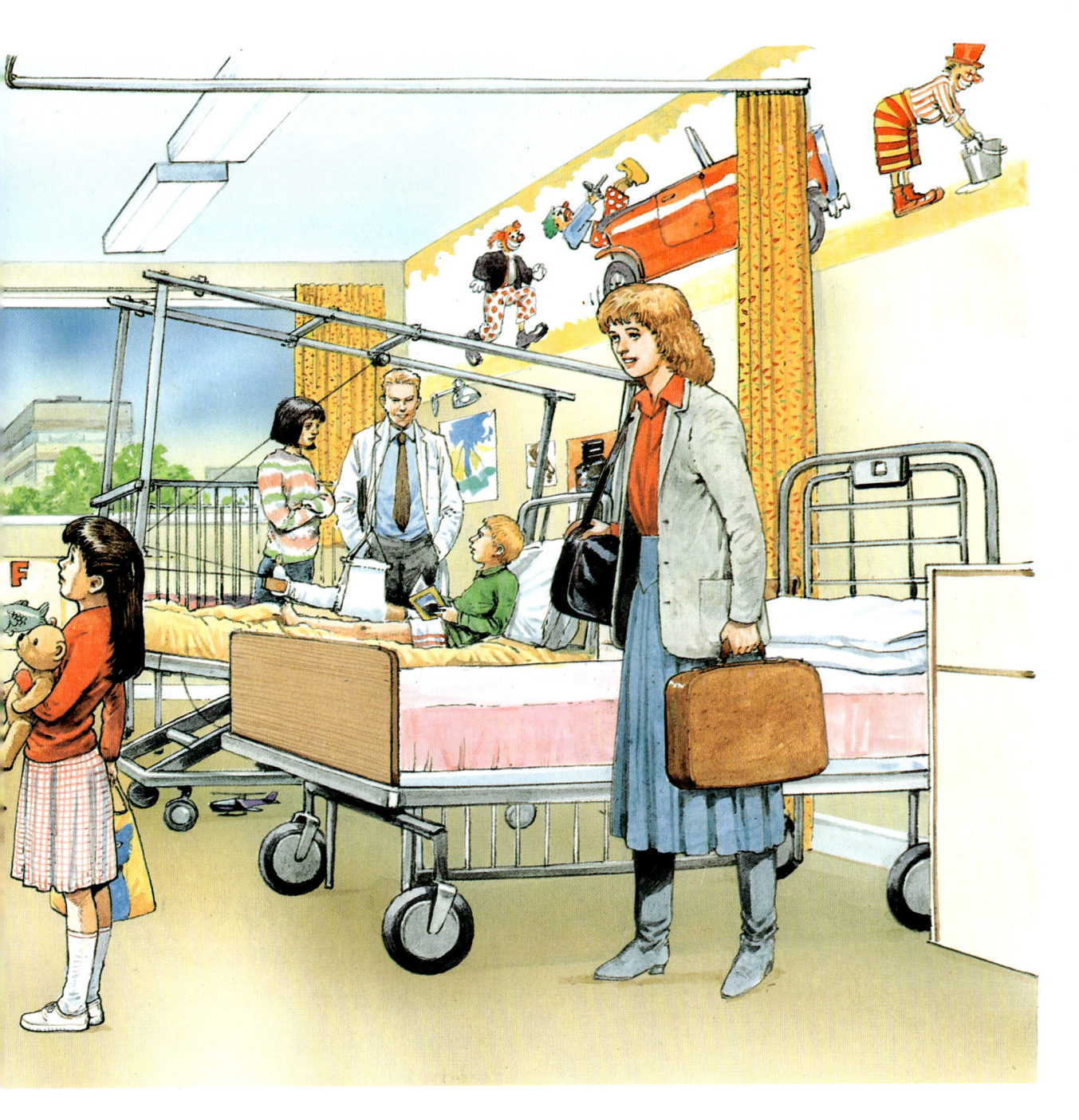

Other nurses work on the Ward too. Helen is a staff nurse. She takes Amy's temperature with a thermometer to measure how hot her body is. She holds Amy's wrist and counts her pulse. The pulse is the throbbing beat you can feel on the inside of your wrist.

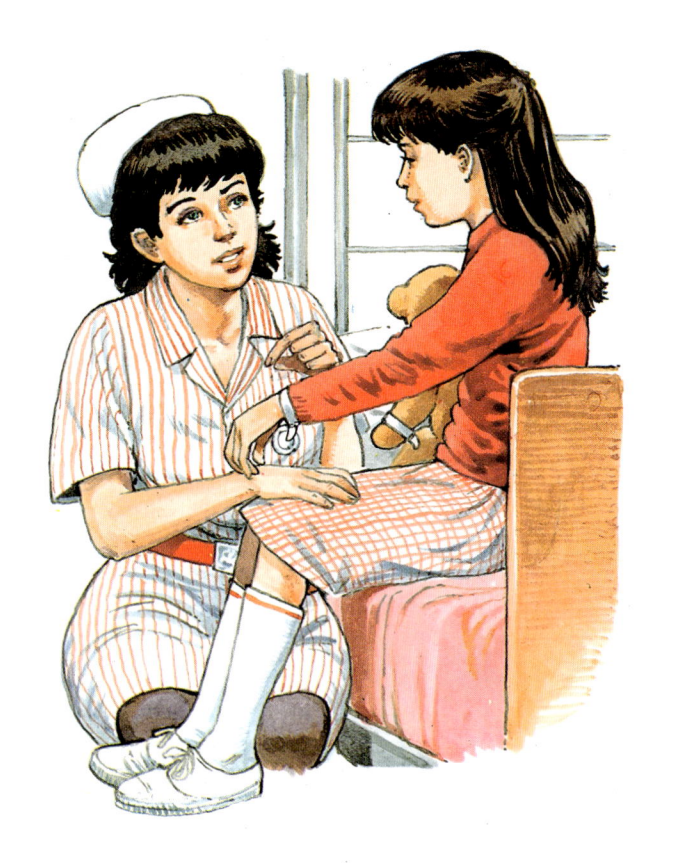

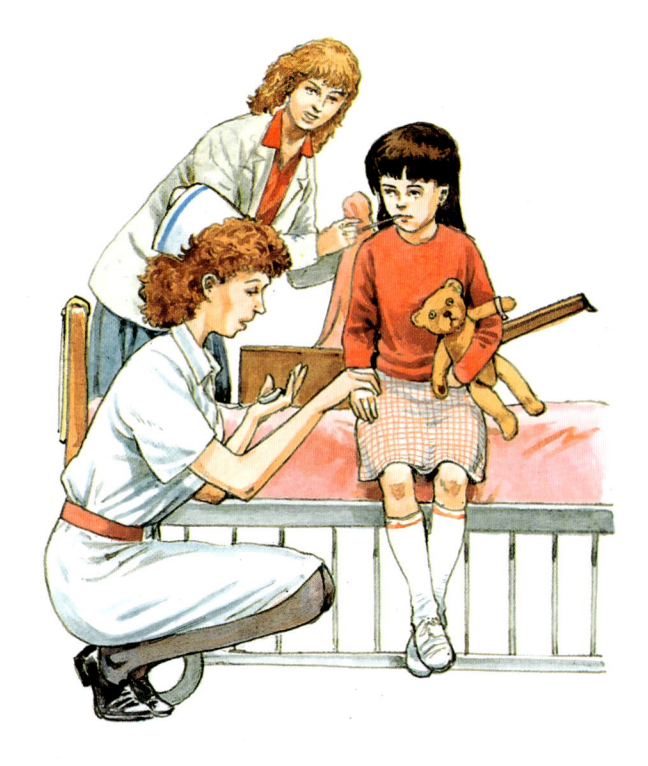

Amy's Mum unpacks Amy's clothes and toys. She is staying with Amy in the hospital.

Marie is still learning how to take care of patients. She is a student nurse. She writes Amy's name on a tag and fixes it around Amy's wrist. Amy's teddy gets a name tag too.

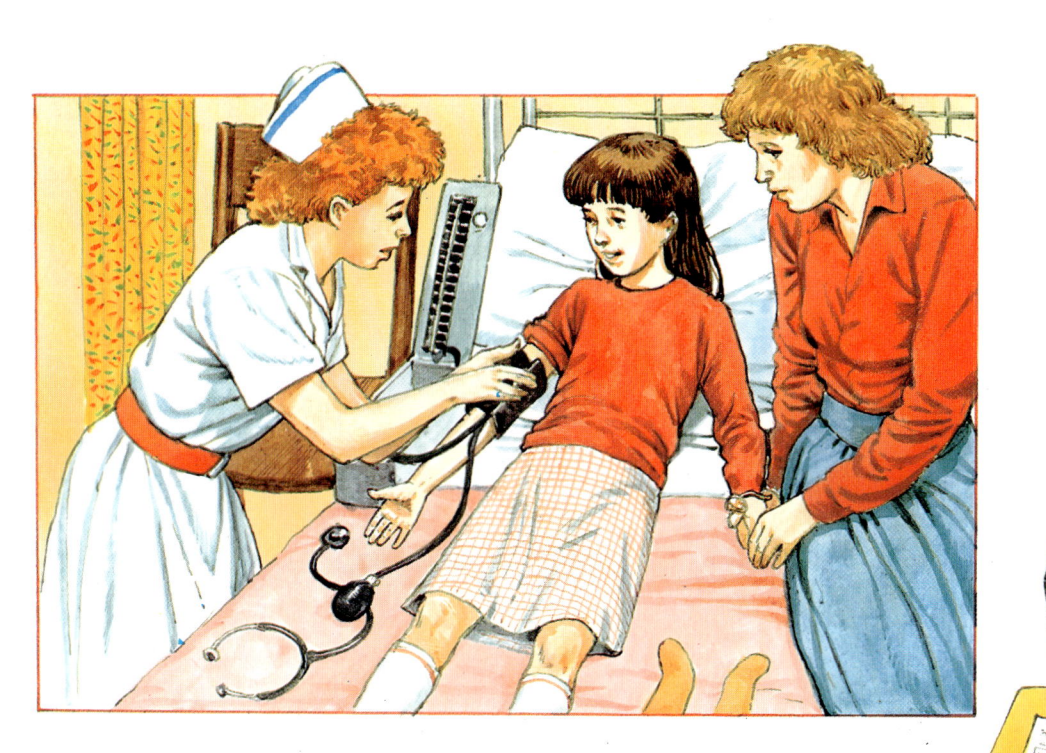

Nurse Helen takes Amy's blood pressure too. She wraps a cuff around Amy's arm and pumps air into it. An instrument connected to the cuff shows how fast Amy's blood is moving.

Helen writes down all the measurements on Amy's chart. The nurses take the measurements of all the children in the Ward at intervals during the day and check the charts to make sure they are getting better.

Cuff

Chart

The instrument which measures blood pressure is a sphygmomanometer.

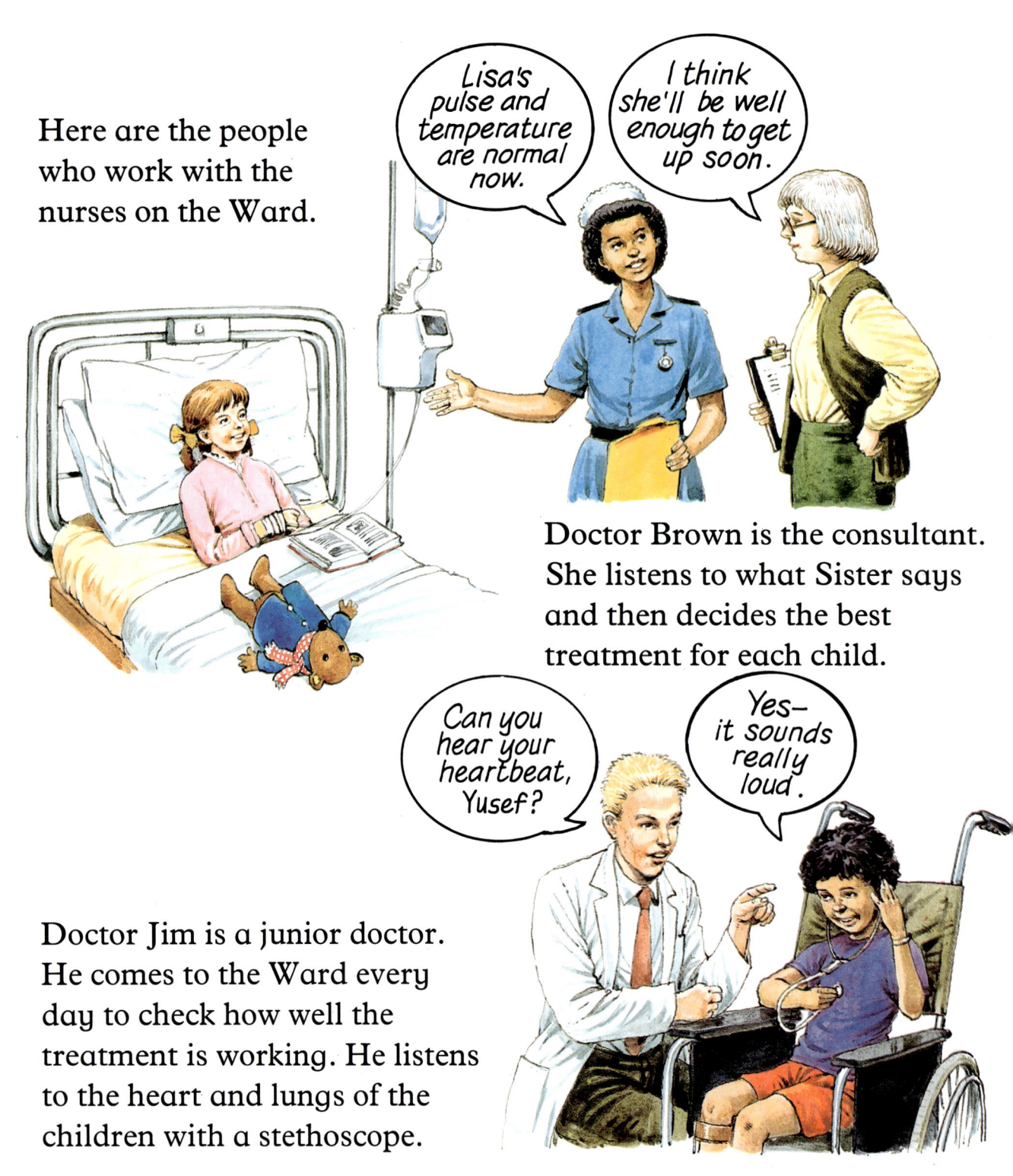

Here are the people who work with the nurses on the Ward.

"Lisa's pulse and temperature are normal now."

"I think she'll be well enough to get up soon."

Doctor Brown is the consultant. She listens to what Sister says and then decides the best treatment for each child.

"Can you hear your heartbeat, Yusef?"

"Yes — it sounds really loud."

Doctor Jim is a junior doctor. He comes to the Ward every day to check how well the treatment is working. He listens to the heart and lungs of the children with a stethoscope.

"How are you today, love?"

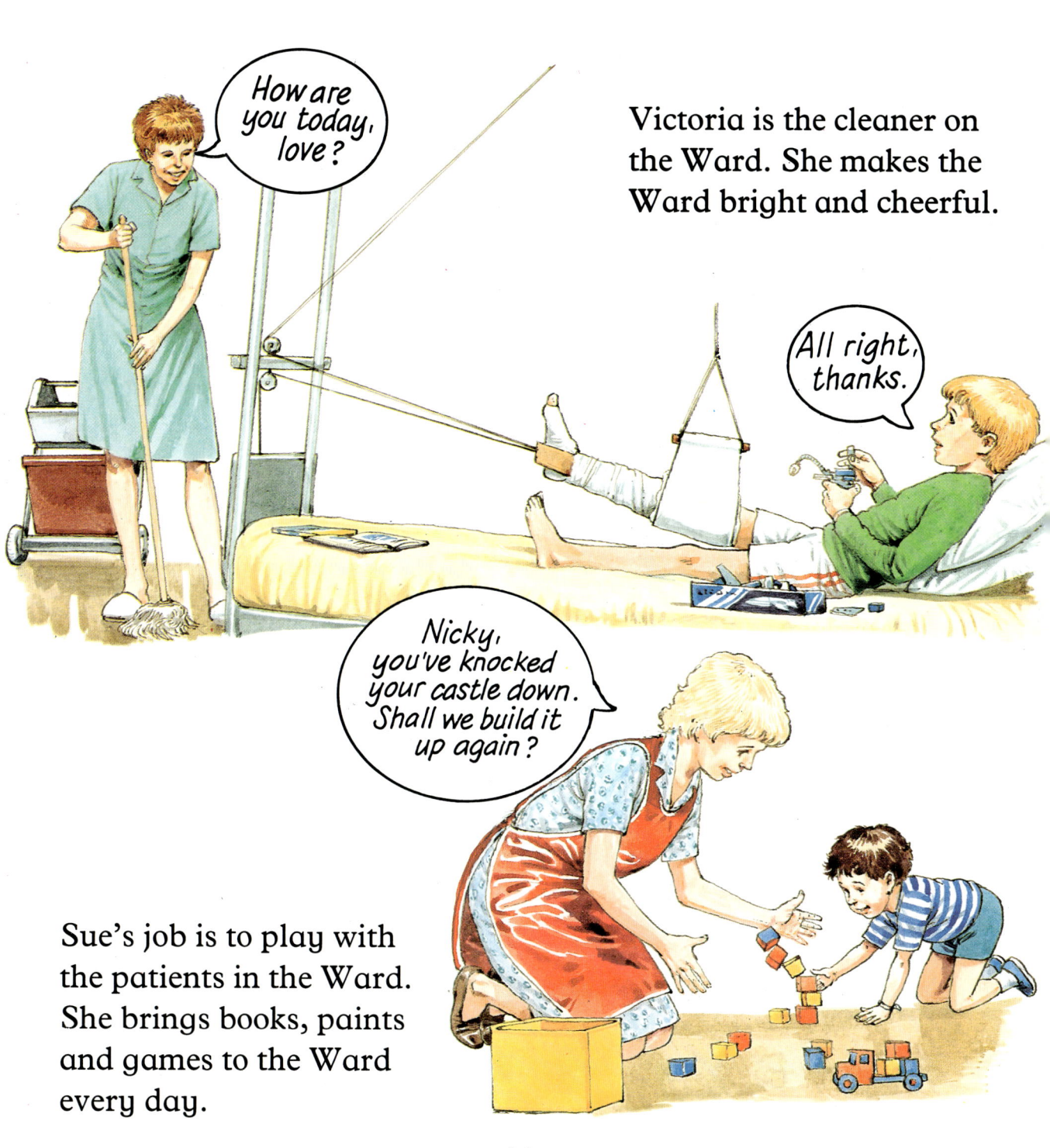

"All right, thanks."

Victoria is the cleaner on the Ward. She makes the Ward bright and cheerful.

"Nicky, you've knocked your castle down. Shall we build it up again?"

Sue's job is to play with the patients in the Ward. She brings books, paints and games to the Ward every day.

The Playroom

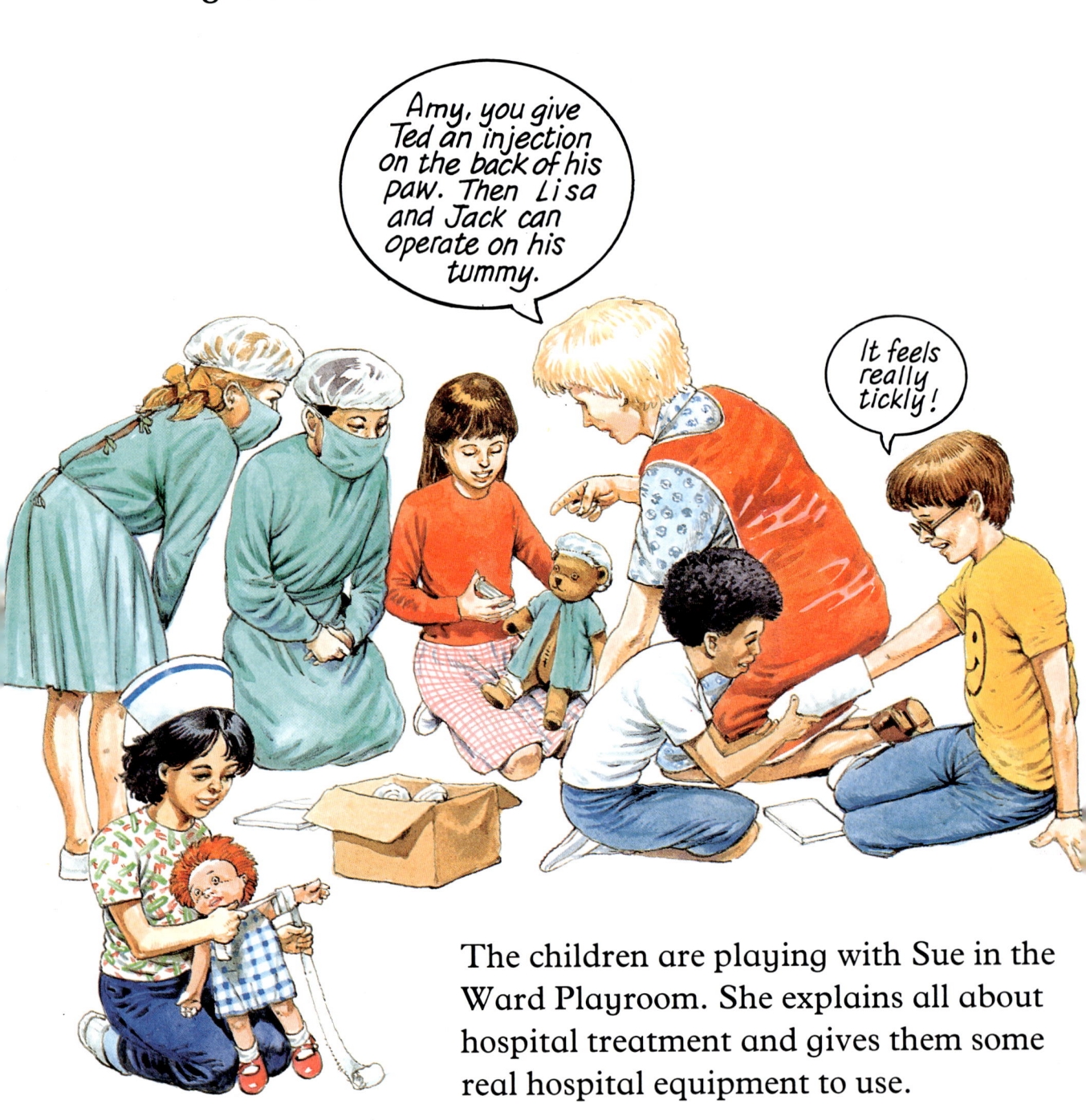

Amy, you give Ted an injection on the back of his paw. Then Lisa and Jack can operate on his tummy.

It feels really tickly!

The children are playing with Sue in the Ward Playroom. She explains all about hospital treatment and gives them some real hospital equipment to use.

Drip — The drip gives Ted a drink.

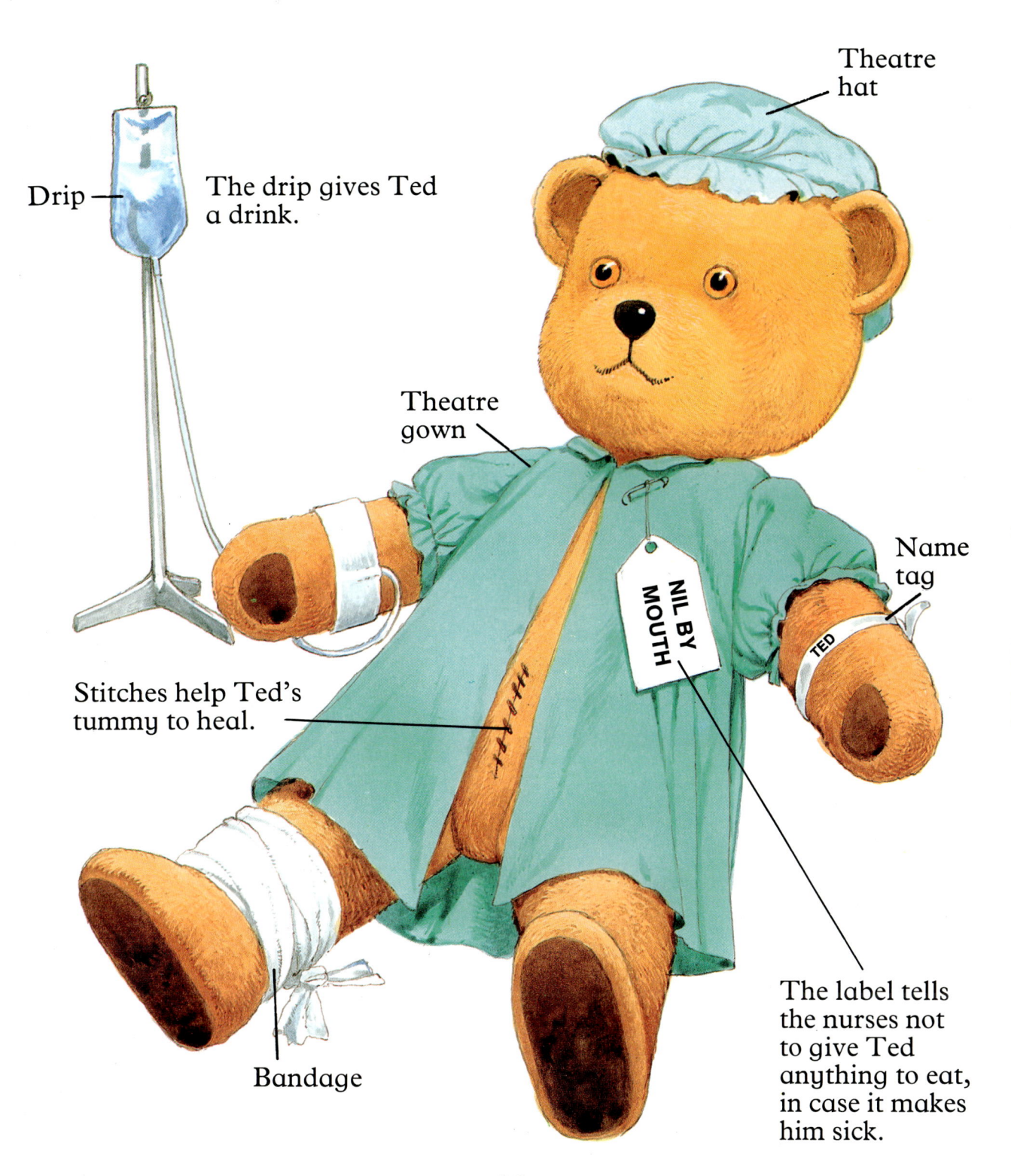

Theatre hat

Theatre gown

Name tag

Stitches help Ted's tummy to heal.

NIL BY MOUTH

The label tells the nurses not to give Ted anything to eat, in case it makes him sick.

Bandage

13

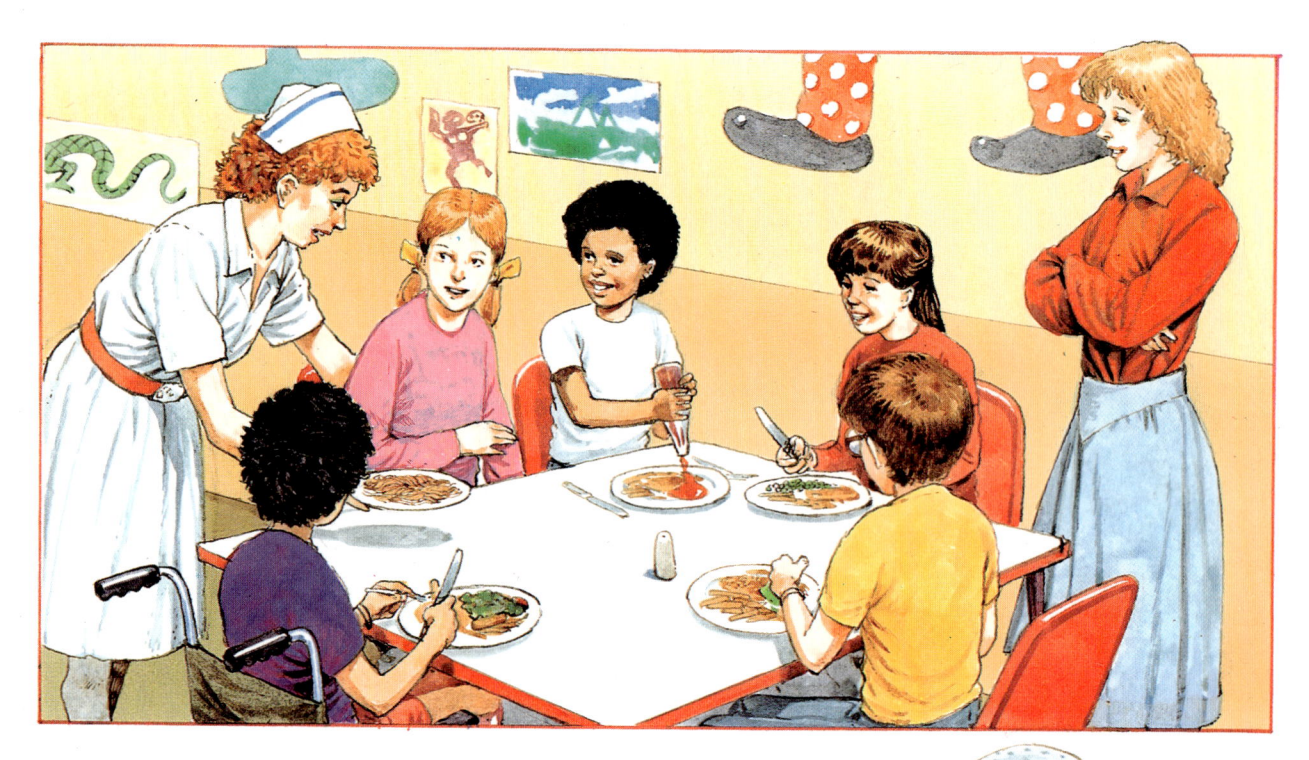

The children eat their meals in the Playroom, unless they have to stay in bed like Martin. The nurses give them their lunch – parents can help too.

"Fish fingers, cheese pie and spaghetti for Robin Ward today."

The kitchens in the hospital are enormous. A team of cooks makes all the meals for the patients. The children choose what they want from a menu.

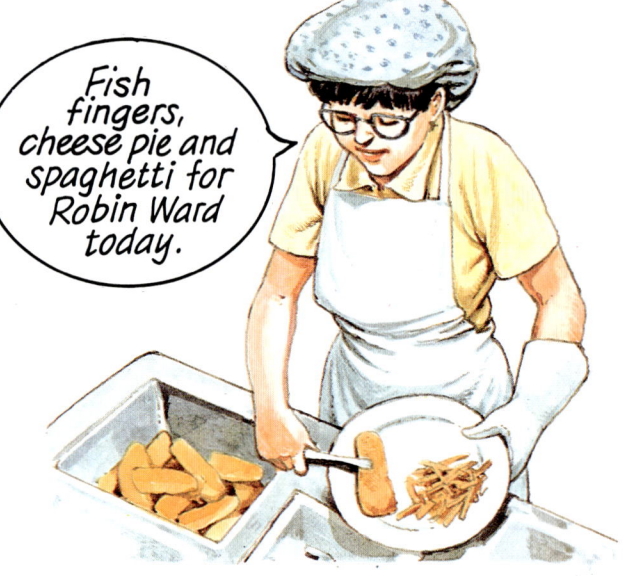

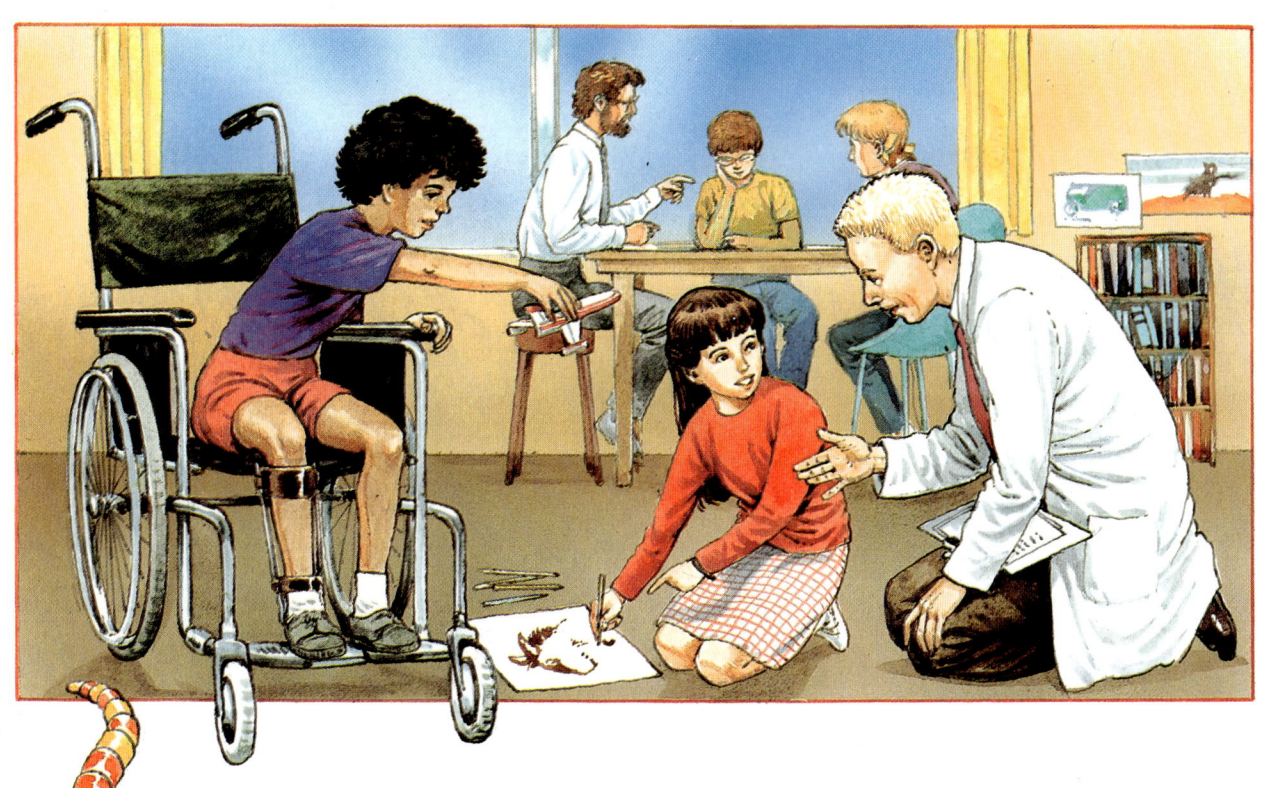

David is the hospital teacher. He brings books and projects for children who have to stay in hospital a long time. Amy will only be in the hospital for two nights so she does not have to work with David unless she wants to.

Doctor Jim comes to tell Amy what will happen during her operation. A doctor called an anaesthetist will make her sleep. Then a doctor called a surgeon will operate on her tummy to repair the hernia.

Amy's Mum can come into the Ward at any time but in the evening Amy's little sister and her Dad come to visit.

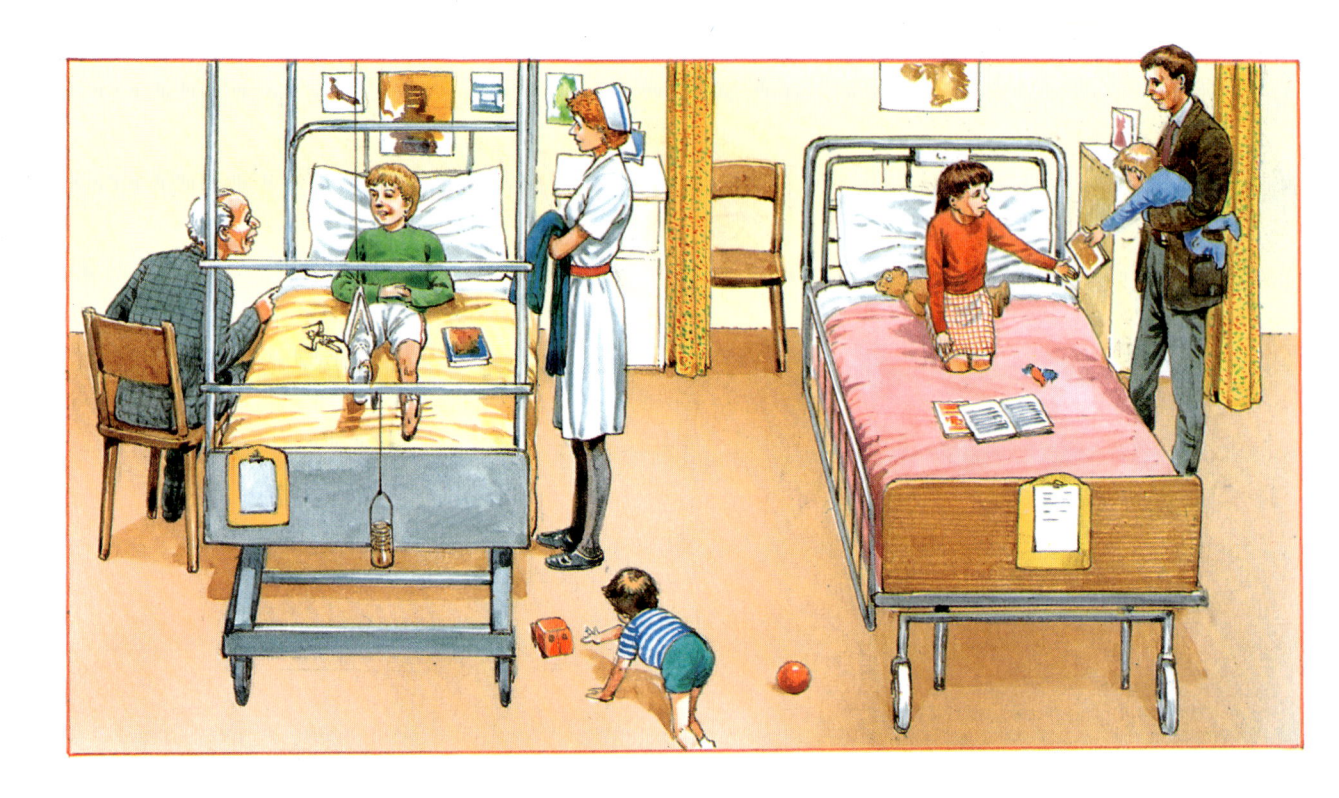

Then it is Amy's bedtime. Amy thinks her bed feels strange but her Mum sits beside her and she soon goes to sleep. Her Mum will sleep nearby. A night nurse stays in the Ward all night to make sure the children are sleeping peacefully. The nurses work in shifts so that there are nurses on duty all the time.

17

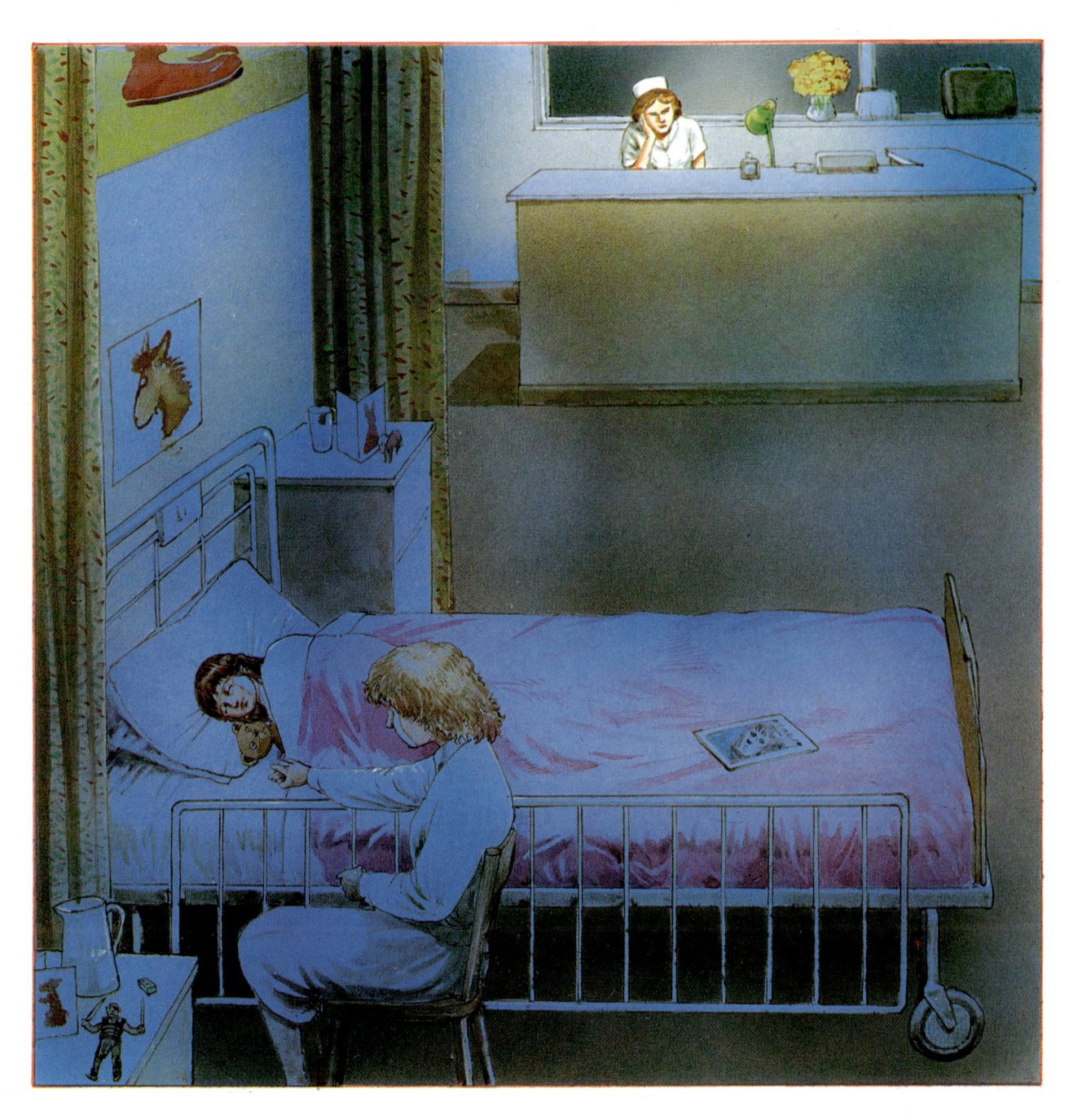

The Hospital at Night

Not everyone in the hospital sleeps at night. In the Maternity Unit tiny babies wake to be fed. In the Intensive Care Ward doctors and nurses work hard all night looking after seriously ill patients. A telephone operator has to keep the telephones working in case there are any emergencies.

The Accident and Emergency Department is often busy. People can have accidents or become ill at any time of the day or night and must be rushed to hospital. If there is a real emergency an ambulance goes off at top speed to fetch the patient. The driver speaks to the hospital by radio so a nurse is waiting to help when they arrive with the new patient.

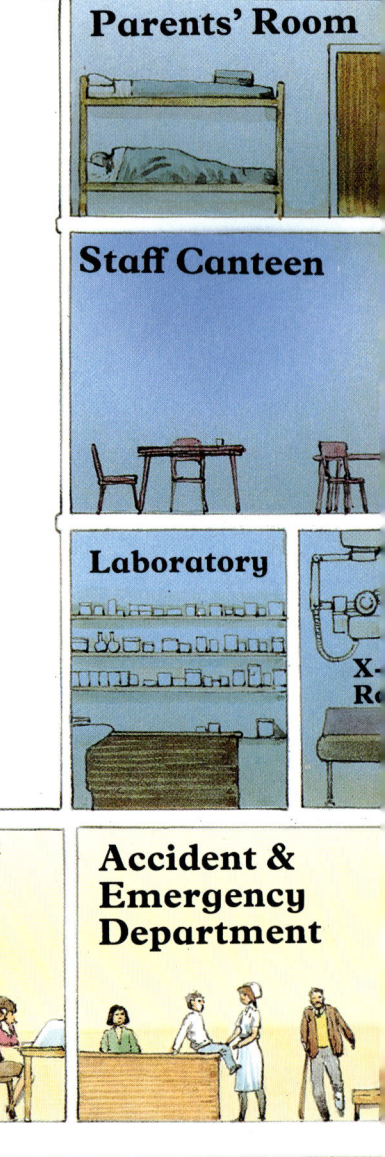

Playroom

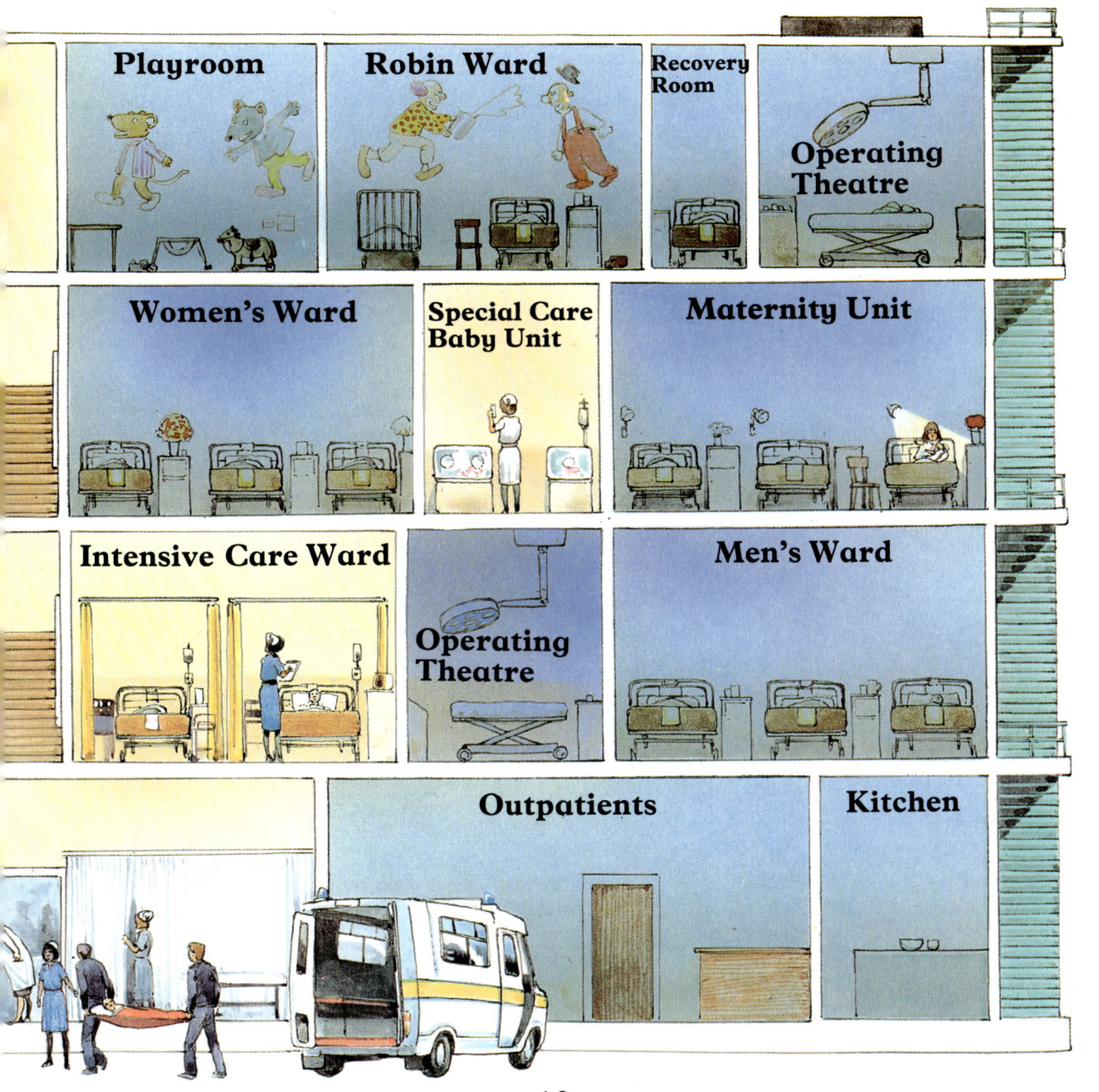

Robin Ward

Recovery Room

Operating Theatre

Women's Ward

Special Care Baby Unit

Maternity Unit

Intensive Care Ward

Operating Theatre

Men's Ward

Outpatients

Kitchen

Ambulance

The Operation

In the morning Amy isn't allowed any breakfast in case it makes her sick while she is in the Operating Theatre.

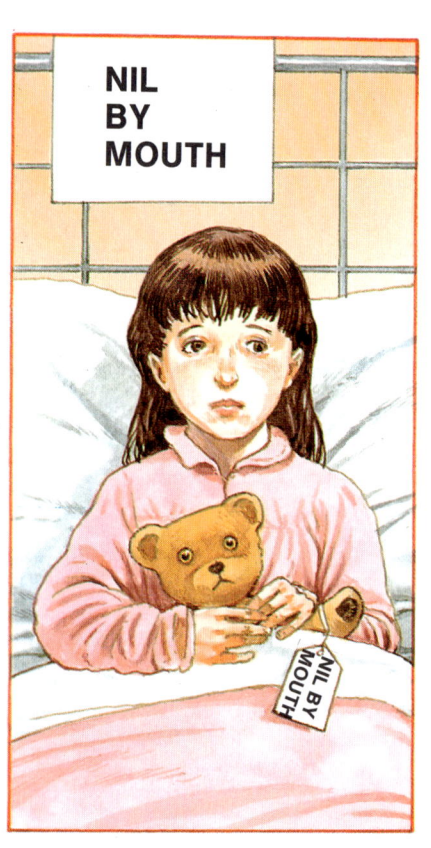

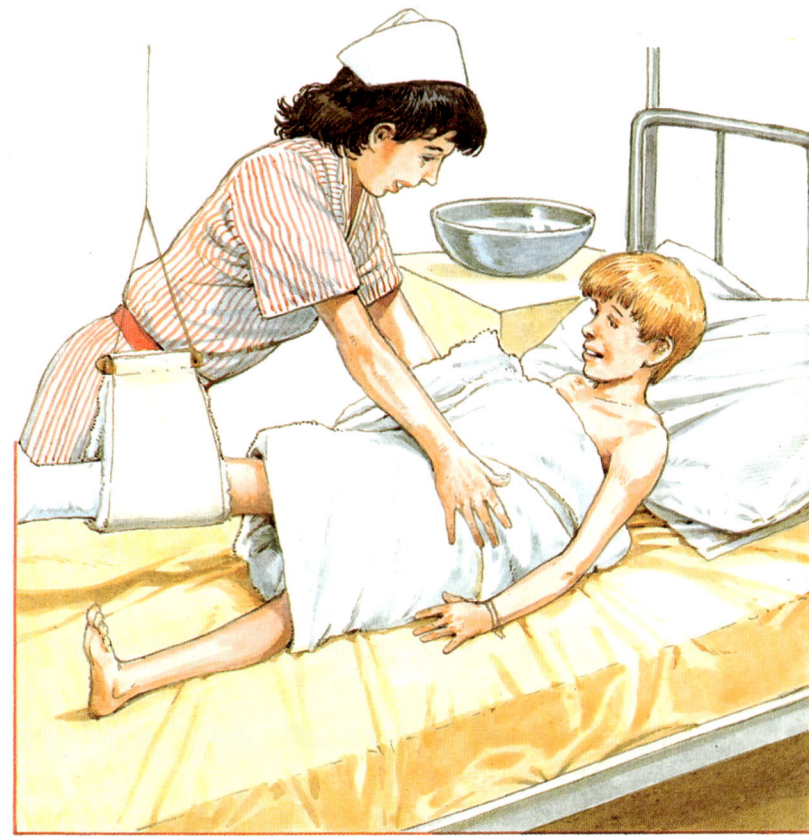

The nurses make the beds and make sure all the children wash. Martin can't go to the bathroom so Nurse Marie gives him a blanket bath. She covers him with towels and washes him bit by bit.

Now Amy is dressed in a theatre gown and hat, ready for her operation. Sister has given her a drink which will start to make her sleepy. Amy gives her teddy a drink too. She tells Sister that he is feeling sleepy.

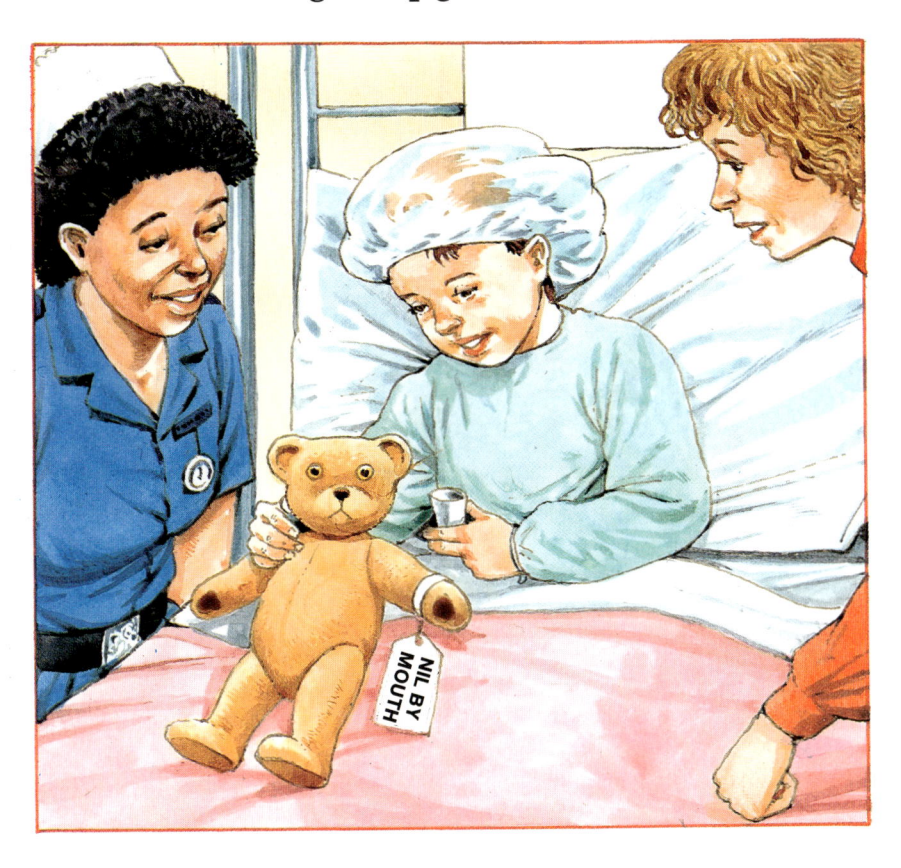

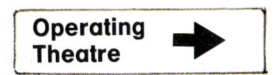

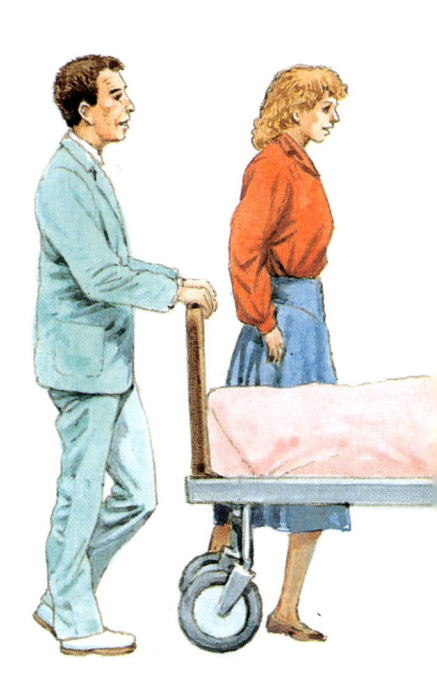

A porter wheels Amy out of the Ward on her bed, and along to the Operating Theatre. Amy's Mum and Nurse Helen come with her.

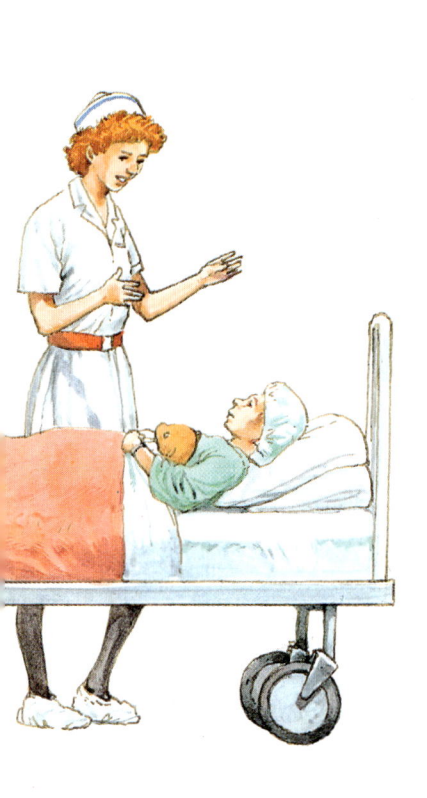

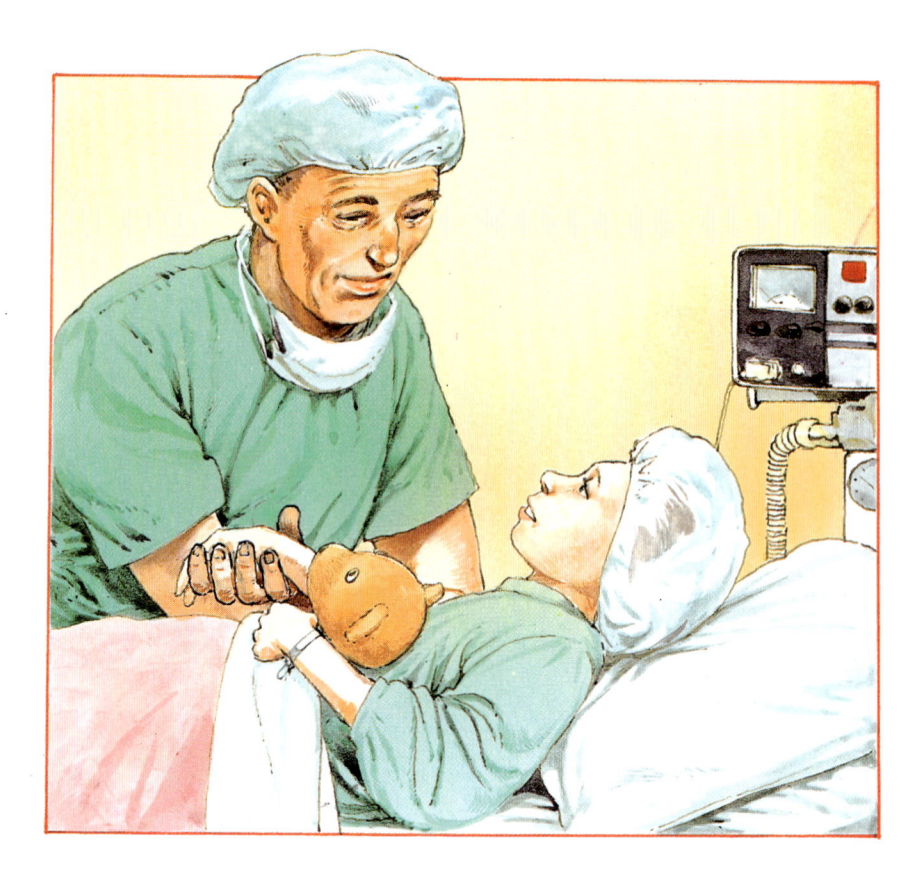

Nurse Helen goes with Amy into the Anaesthetics Room. By this time Amy is very sleepy. The anaesthetist explains that he will send her into a special kind of sleep. It is called anaesthesia. This means that the patient doesn't feel anything during the operation. The anaesthetist will stay with her all through the operation, checking her pulse and her breathing. After the operation she will wake up.

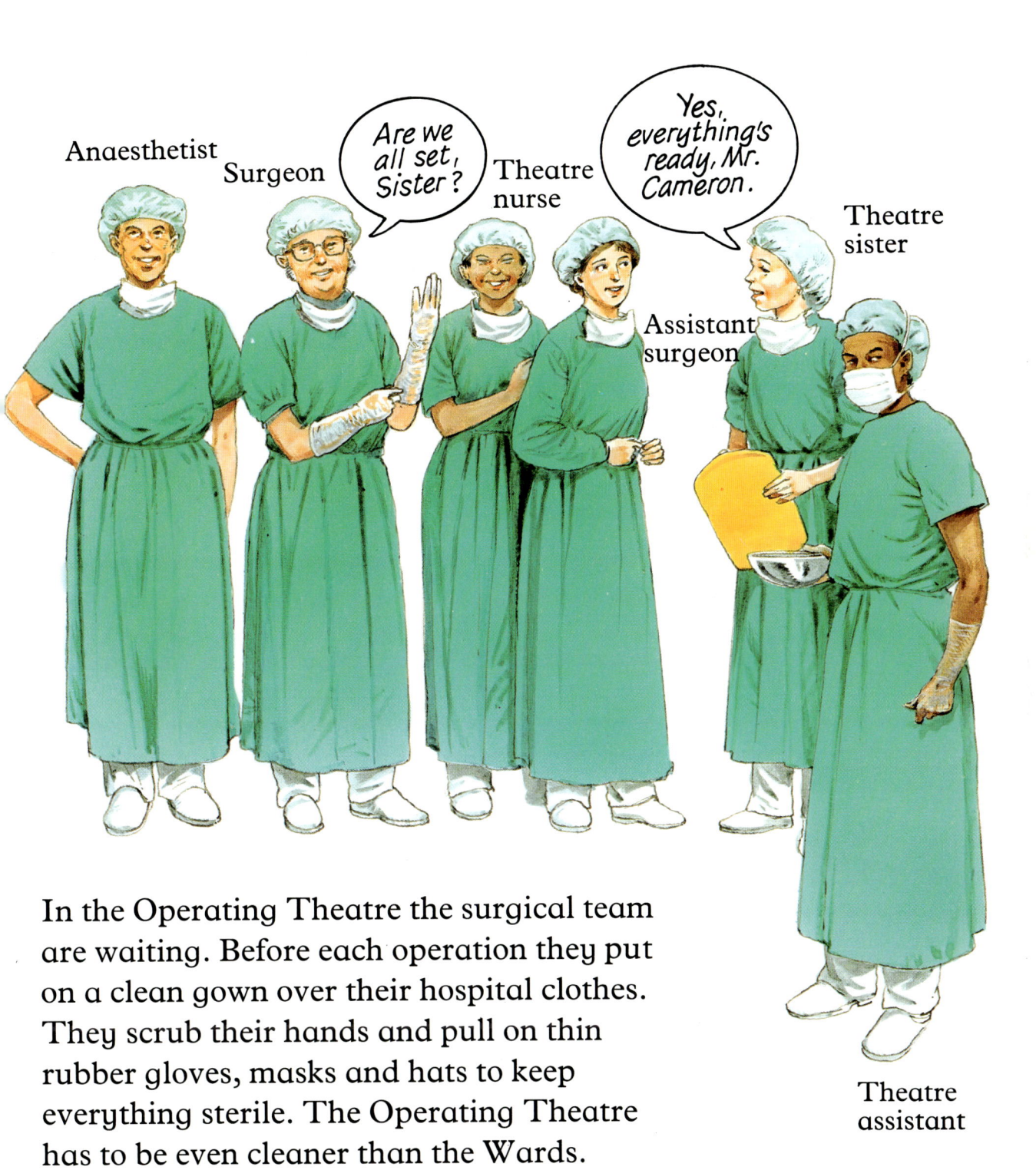

Anaesthetist

Surgeon

"Are we all set, Sister?"

Theatre nurse

"Yes, everything's ready, Mr. Cameron."

Theatre sister

Assistant surgeon

Theatre assistant

In the Operating Theatre the surgical team are waiting. Before each operation they put on a clean gown over their hospital clothes. They scrub their hands and pull on thin rubber gloves, masks and hats to keep everything sterile. The Operating Theatre has to be even cleaner than the Wards.

After the operation Amy is taken into the Recovery Room where she wakes up. She is still very sleepy because of the anaesthetic. Then a porter wheels her back to the Ward. The first person she sees when she wakes up again is her Mum.

The nurses are as busy as ever but Sister Carole stops to say hello. She and Nurse Marie are taking the medicine trolley around the Ward. Sister will look at the charts on the end of each bed to see what kind of medicine the doctors have written down for each patient. Some children can drink their medicine. Others swallow pills.

The physiotherapist is teaching Martin some exercises to keep his left leg strong while his broken leg mends.

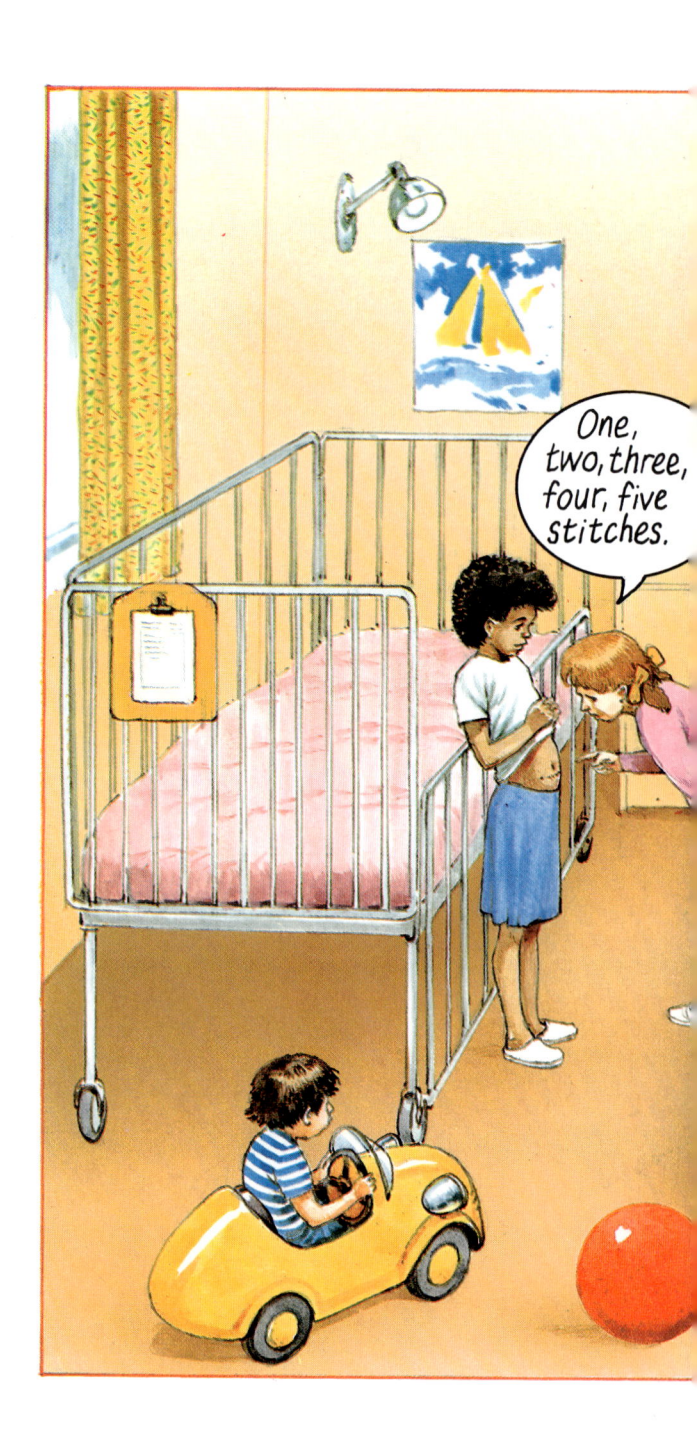

25

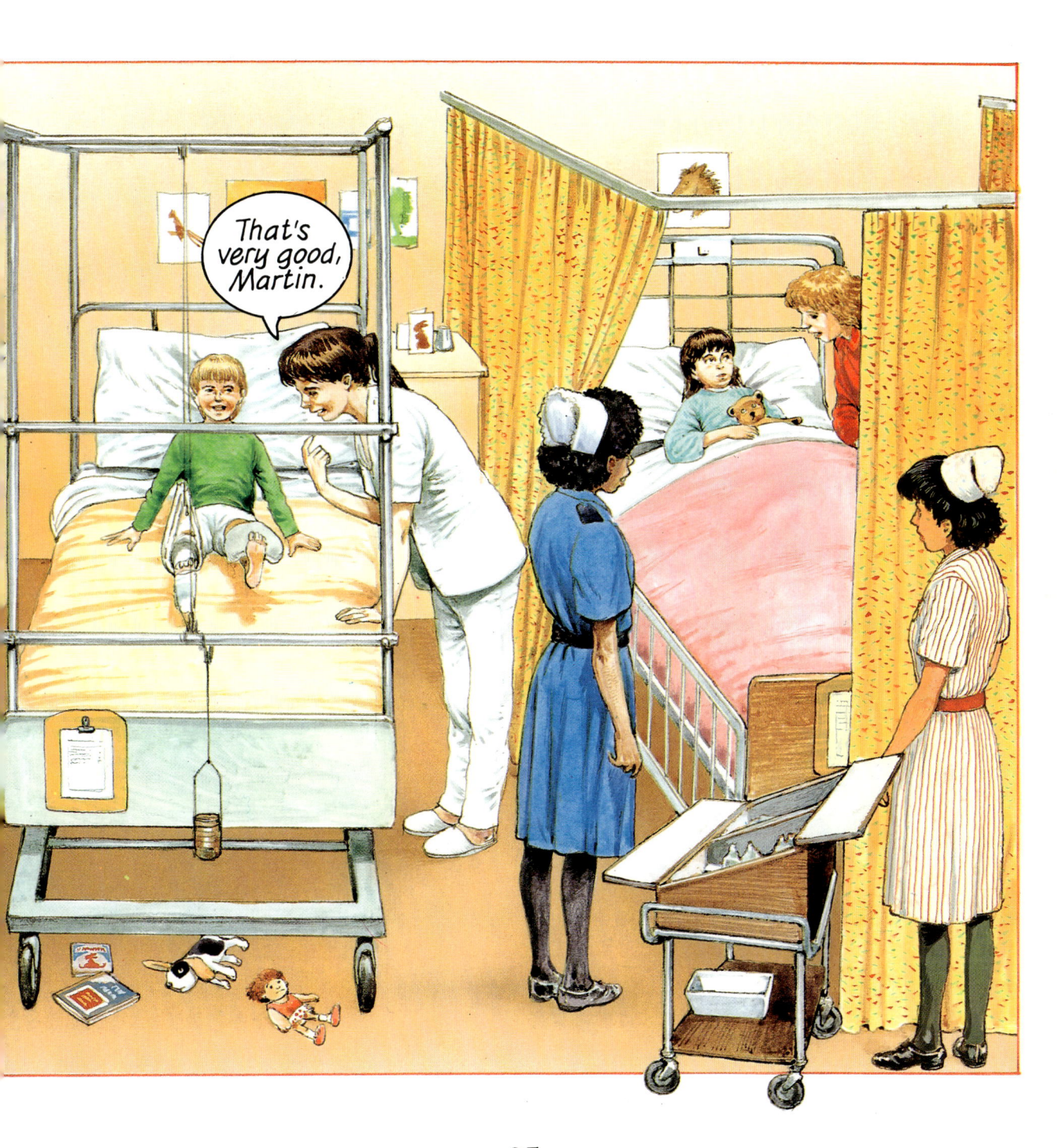

Next morning Amy asks for a big breakfast. She is very hungry even though her tummy is a little sore. Doctor Jim comes to see how she is feeling. He says that Amy is well enough to go home later today.

Amy has stayed two nights in hospital but many children come just to have treatment and then go home straight away.

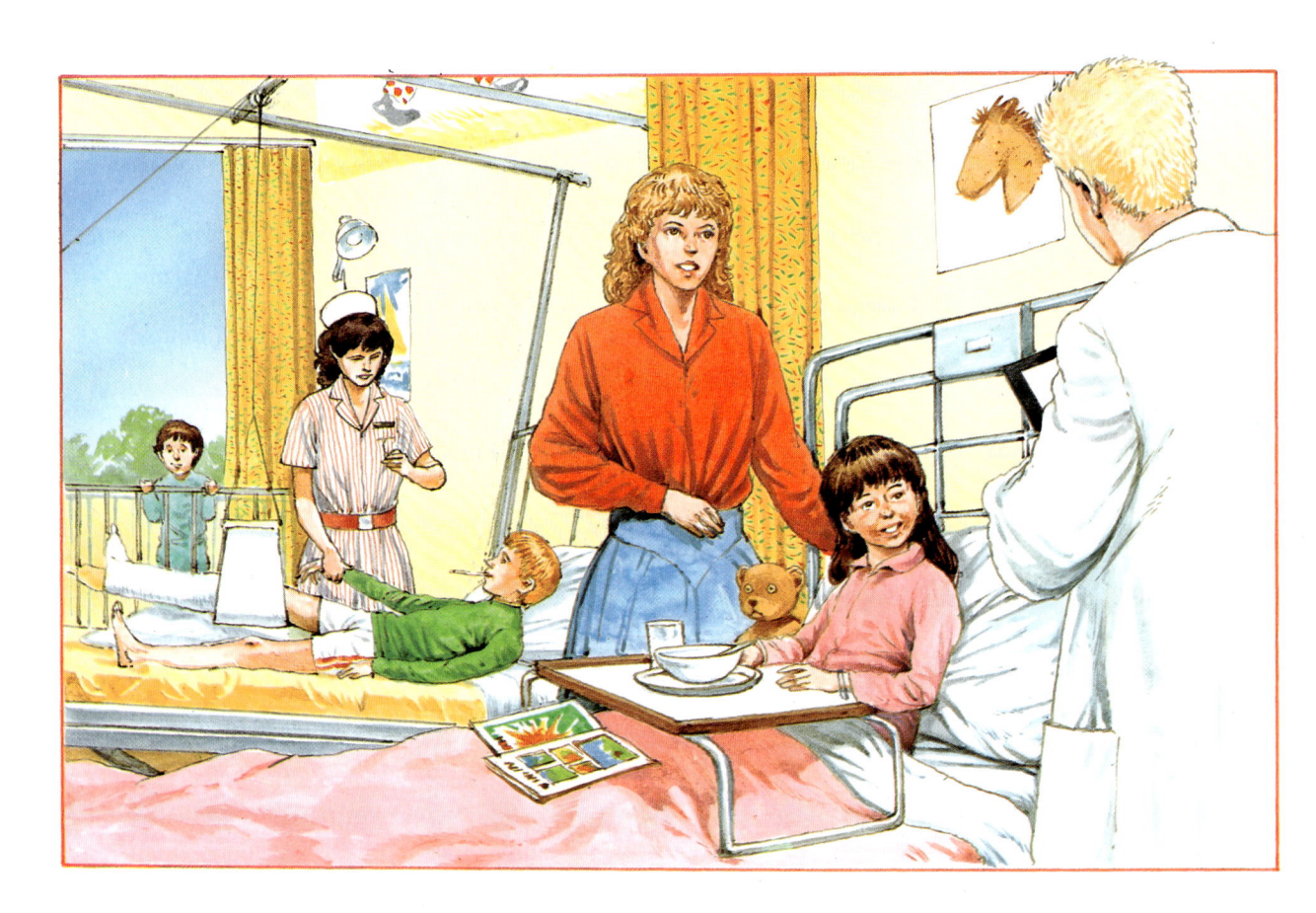

Accident & Emergency

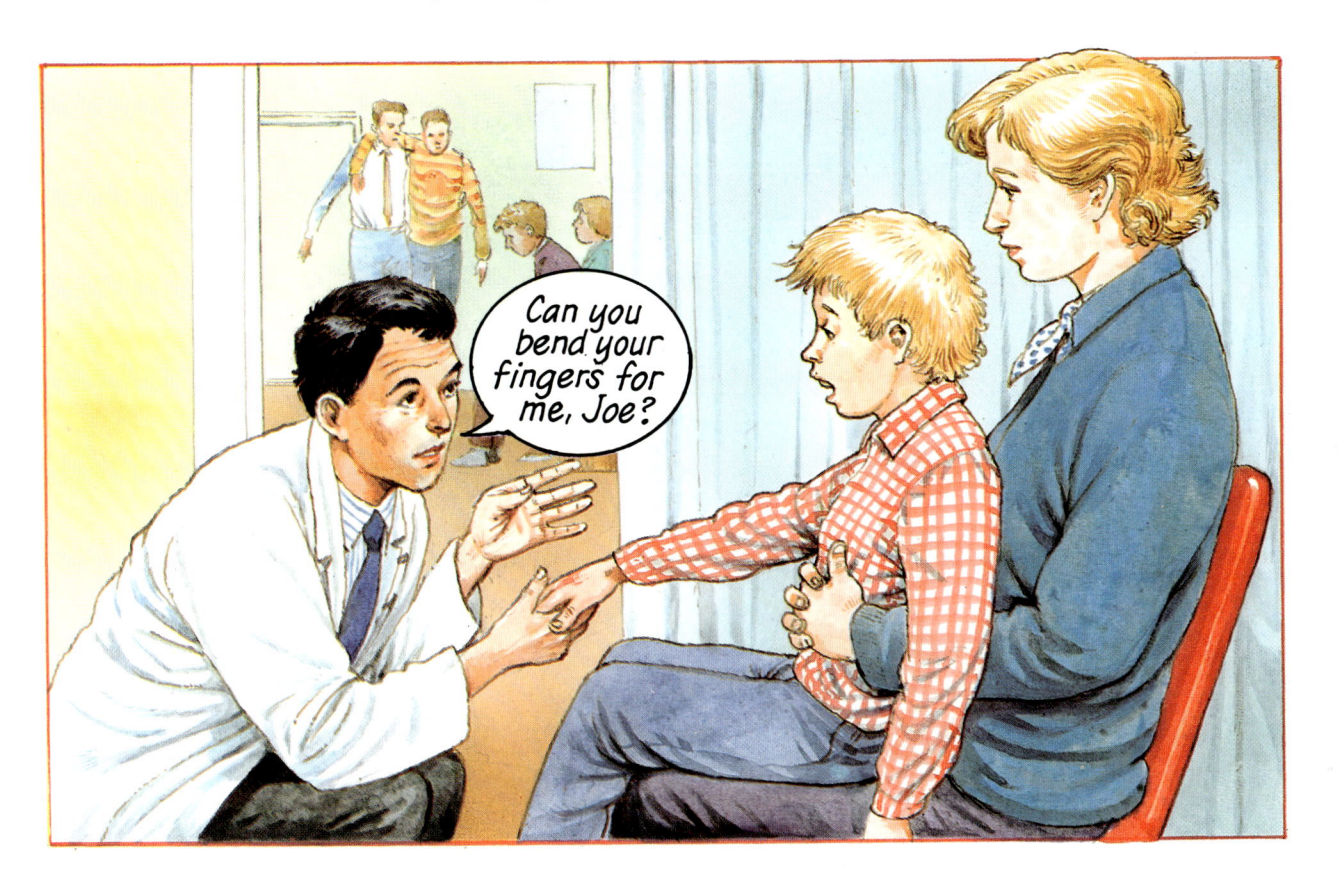

Joe fell off a climbing frame this morning. His hand is painful and a little bit swollen. So his mother has brought him to the Accident and Emergency Department. First they speak to the receptionist.

Then Doctor Paul examines Joe's hand. He decides that Joe should have an X-ray to make sure no bones have been broken.

An X-ray

In the X-ray Room the radiographer pulls down the big X-ray camera over Joe's hand. Then she stands behind a screen, and presses a button to take the picture. Her job is to use the X-ray machine to take different kinds of pictures of people's insides which will help doctors to understand what is wrong with their patients. Technicians develop the X-ray film just like a photograph taken by an ordinary camera.

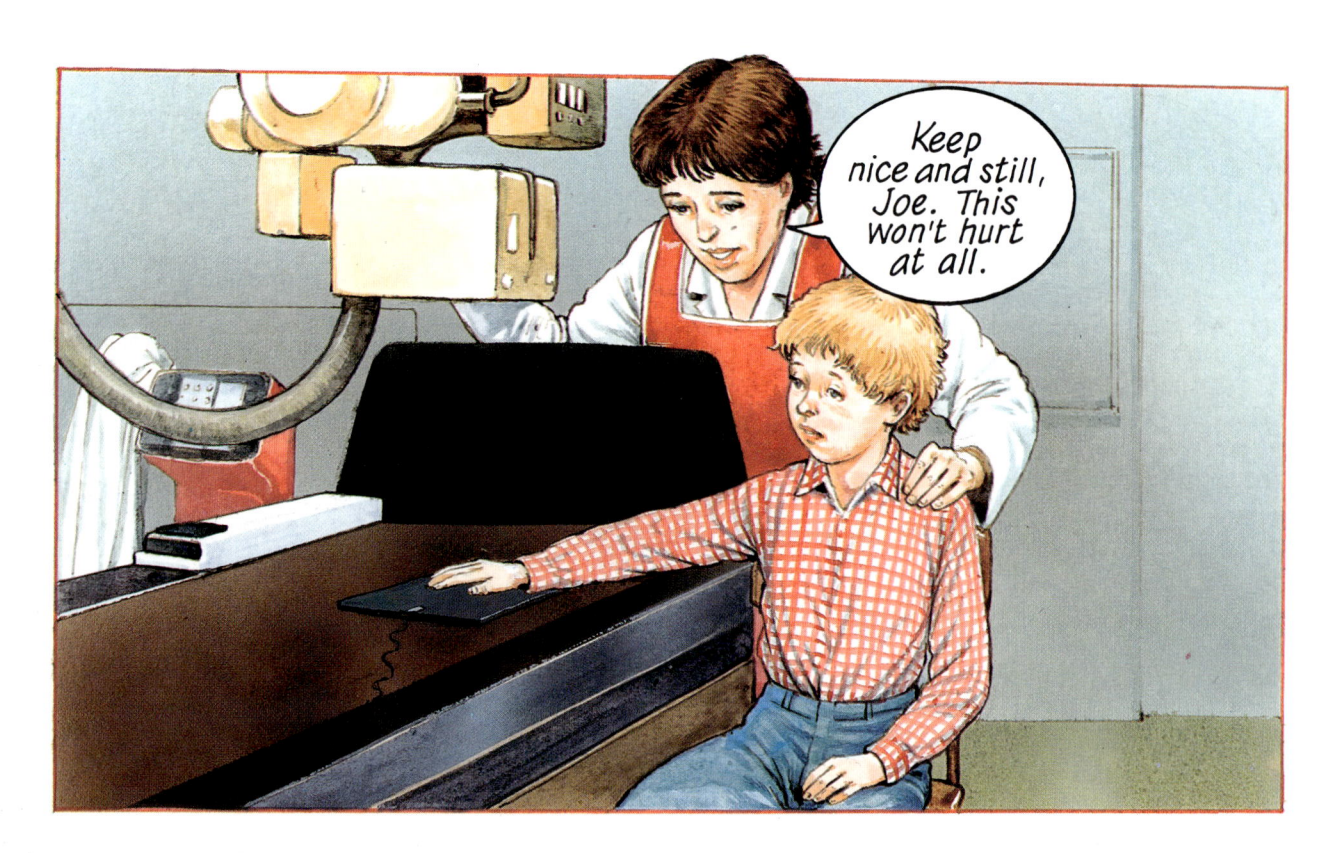

Doctor Paul, Joe and his mother look at the X-ray picture. Good news – none of the bones is broken. Joe's hand is sore because he bruised it badly when he fell to the ground. It will soon get better.

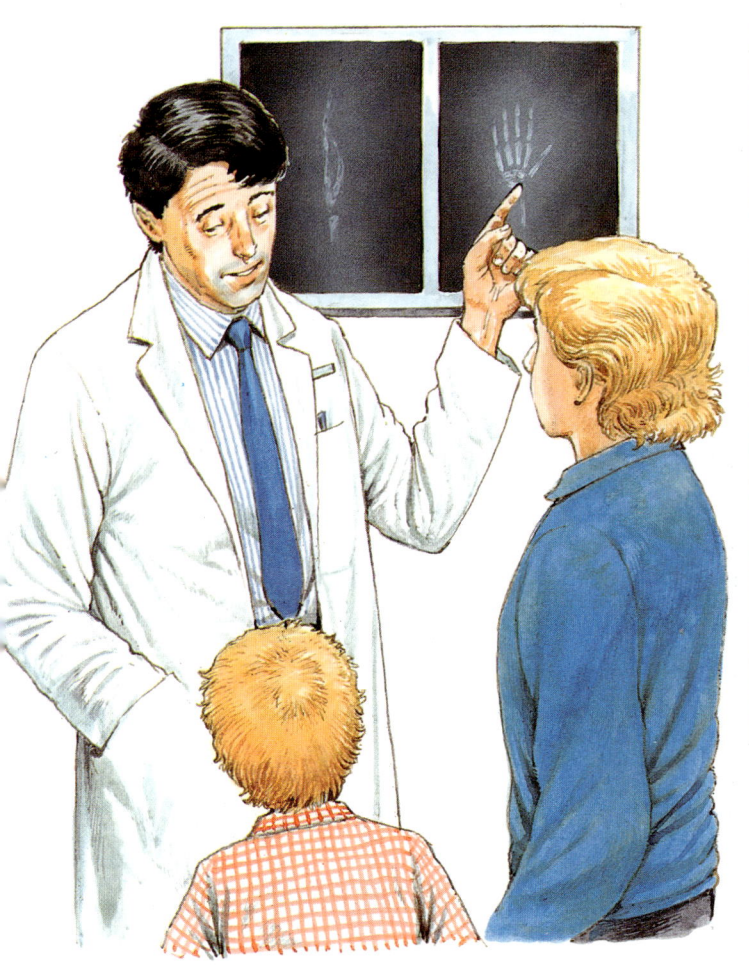

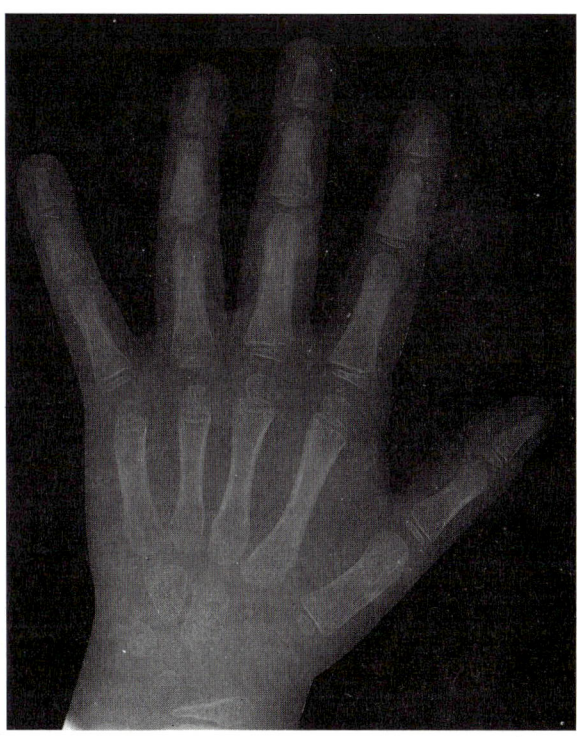

This X-ray shows all the bones inside a hand. None of them is broken.

Nurse Kevin puts a dressing on Joe's hand to keep it clean and winds a bandage on top to protect it.

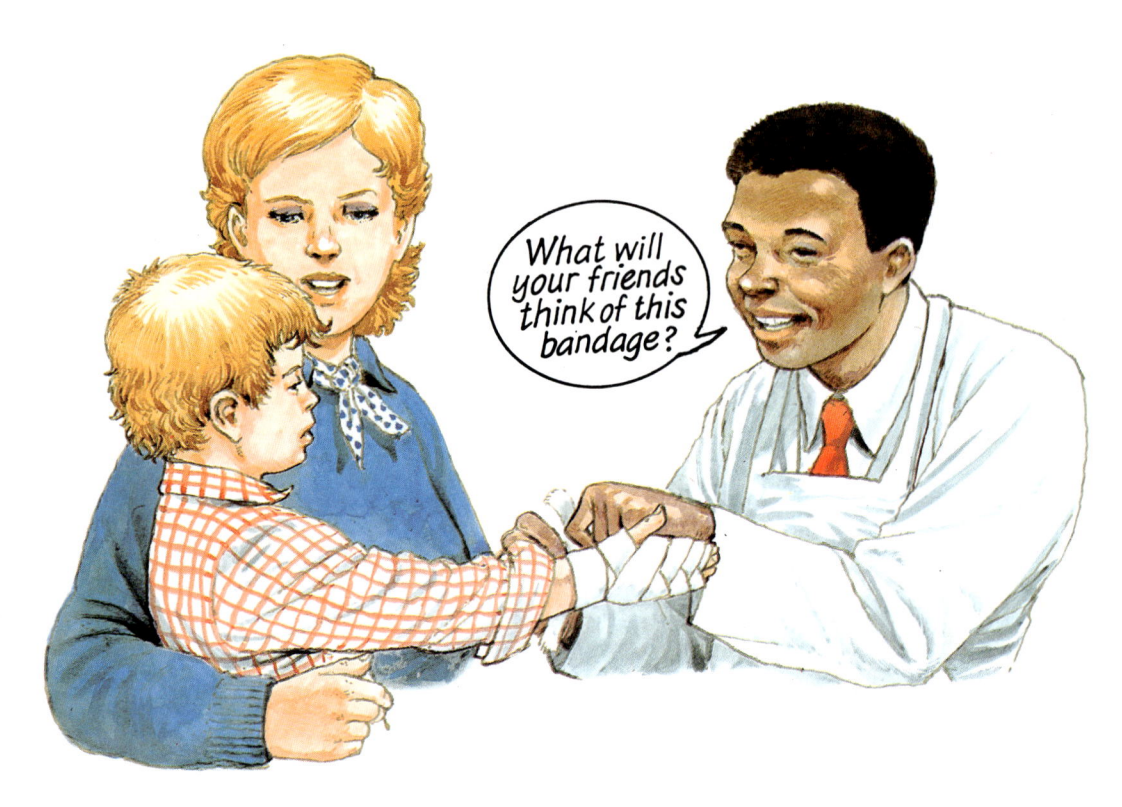

What will your friends think of this bandage?

Amy and Joe can both go home now but the hospital is still busy. More patients are arriving all the time. The nurses and doctors and all the other hospital workers will always be there, ready to take care of people when they are ill.

◀ Accident & Emergency

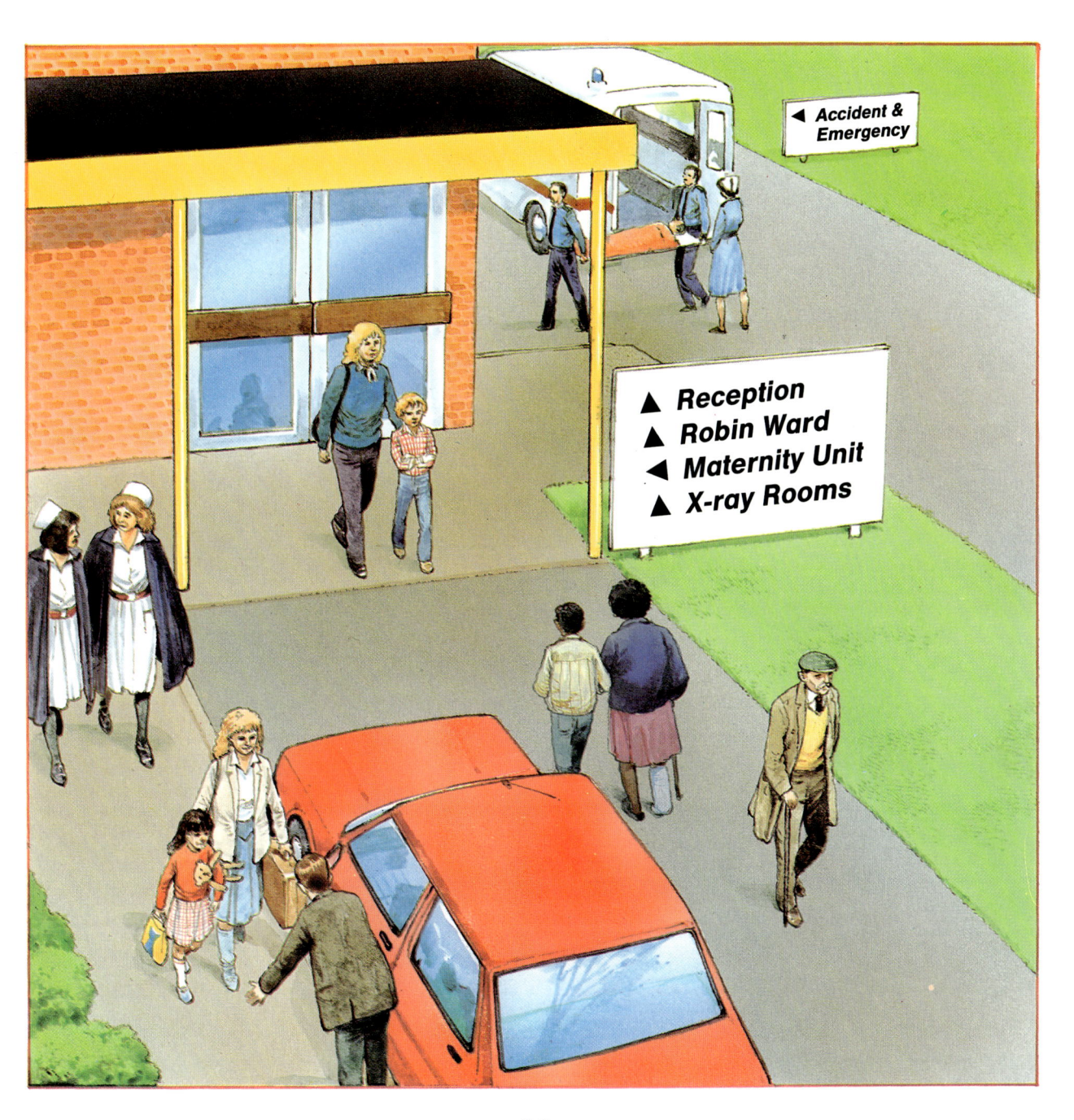

▲ Reception
▲ Robin Ward
◀ Maternity Unit
▲ X-ray Rooms

Index

Accident and Emergency 4, 5, 18, 27
ambulance 18, 19
ambulance driver 18, 19
anaesthetist 15, 22, 23

bandage 13, 30
blanket bath 20
blood pressure 9

chart 9, 24
cleaners 11
consultant 10
cooks 14

doctors 4, 10, 15, 18, 23, 24, 26, 27, 28, 29, 30
drip 13

injection 12
Intensive Care Ward 5, 18, 19

Kitchen 5, 14, 19

Laboratory 4, 18

Maternity Unit 4, 5, 18, 19
meals 14, 20, 26
medicine 24
name tag 8, 13
nurses 4, 6, 8, 9, 10, 14, 16, 18, 20, 21, 22, 23, 24, 30

Operating Theatre 4, 5, 19, 20, 21, 23
operation 4, 6, 13, 15, 21, 22, 23, 24
Outpatients 5, 19

patients 4, 8, 11, 14, 18, 22, 24, 28, 30
physiotherapist 24
Playroom 5, 12, 14, 19
porters 4, 21, 24
pulse 8, 10, 22

radiographer 28
Recovery Room 5, 19, 24

Special Care Baby Unit 5, 19
sphygmomanometer 9
stitches 13, 24
surgeons 15, 23

teacher 15
technicians 28
telephone operator 18
temperature 8, 10
theatre assistant 23
theatre nurse 23
theatre sister 23
thermometer 8

wards 4, 5, 6, 8, 9, 10, 11, 16, 18, 19, 21, 23, 24

X-rays 27, 28, 29
X-ray Room 4, 18, 28

NAWCH (The National Association for the Welfare of Children in Hospital) at Argyle House, 29–31 Euston Road, London NW1 2SD (071 833 2041) is happy to offer information and advice to children going into hospital.

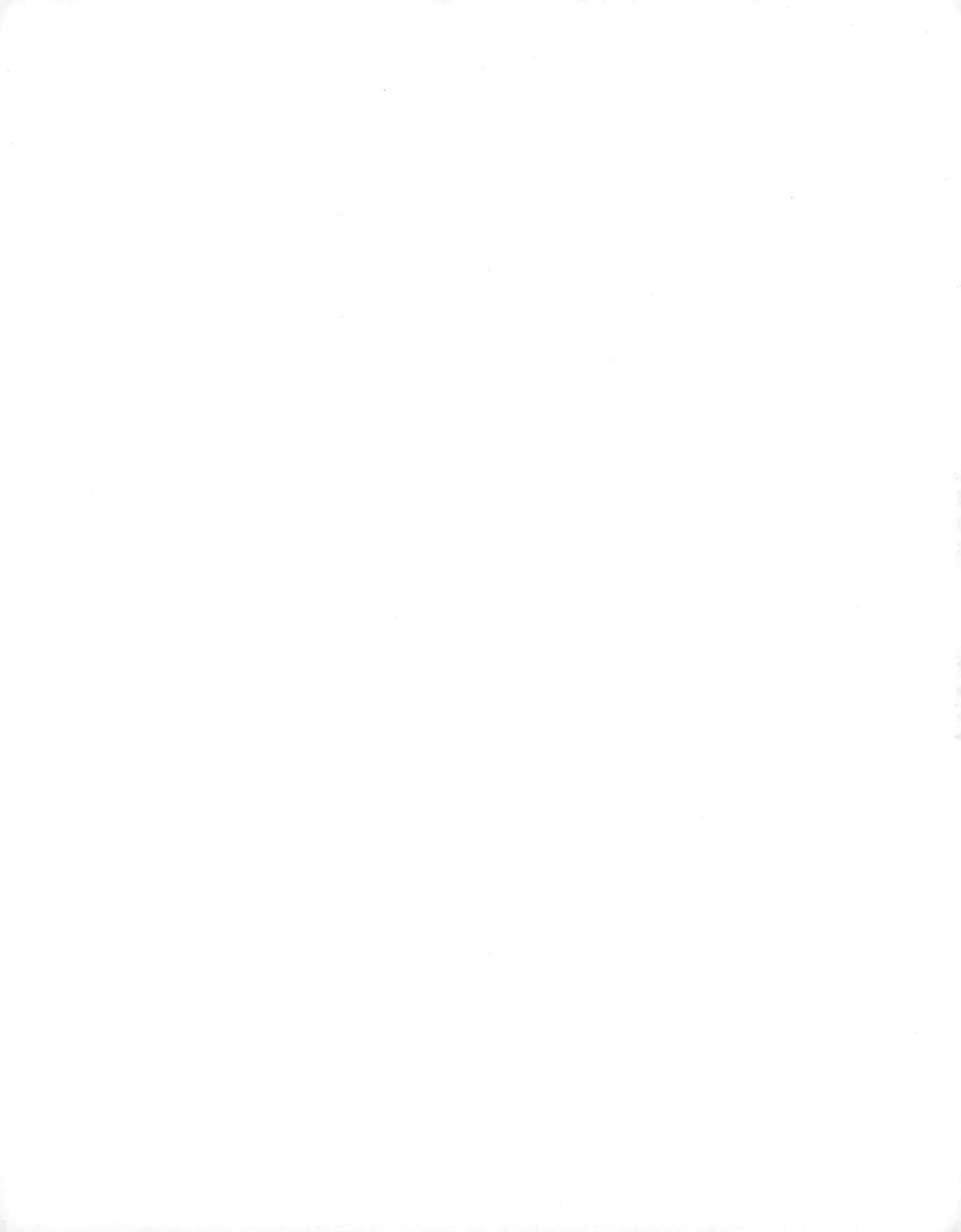